trick
yourself
to
sleep

trick yourself to sleep

222 Ways to Fall and Stay Asleep
from the Science of Slumber

KIM JONES
Foreword by Sarah Brewer, PhD

THE EXPERIMENT

NEW YORK

Contents

Foreword
by Dr. Sarah Brewer

Everyone experiences sleep problems at some time during their life. Often the problems are short-lived, caused by fleeting issues such as jet lag or worry about a job interview or driving test. But sleeplessness that's a result of ongoing problems such as work stress, for instance, may last for weeks and, if not tackled, can become a long-term condition that interferes with your quality of life.

Lack of sleep is also bad for your health. Research consistently shows that people who sleep soundly for seven to eight hours at a time have the lowest risk of high blood pressure, heart disease, depression, and obesity, and also mount better immune responses against infection.[1]

Adequate sleep may even help you live longer, if a study that followed twenty-one thousand sets of twins for over twenty-two years is to be believed. According to the results, those who achieved the magic seven to eight hours' sleep per night lived longer than those who habitually slept for shorter or longer periods.

If sleep eludes you, sleeping pills are not the answer. Instead, follow the advice in this fabulous book and tackle your sleep problems naturally using diet, lifestyle, cognitive, mindful, and other alternative approaches. You'll be glad to know that doesn't include the proverbial counting of sheep—far too boring an exercise to distract you from your genuine worries.

I can guarantee you will find numerous sleep-inducing suggestions you've never encountered before, at least one of which is bound to work for you.

DR. SARAH BREWER,
MSc (NutrMed), MA (Cantab), MB, BChir,
RNutr, MBANT, CNHC
DrSarahBrewer.com

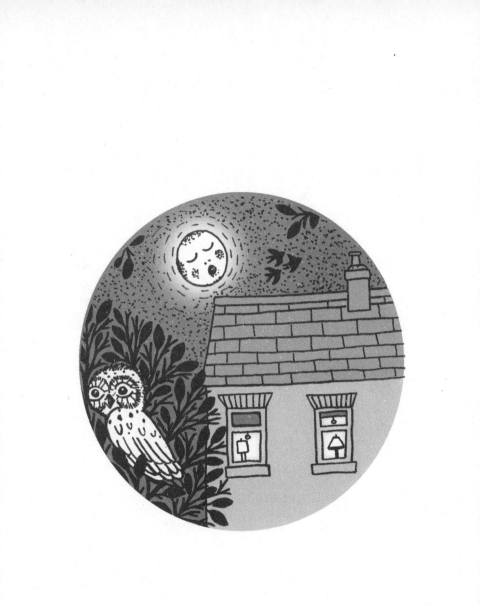

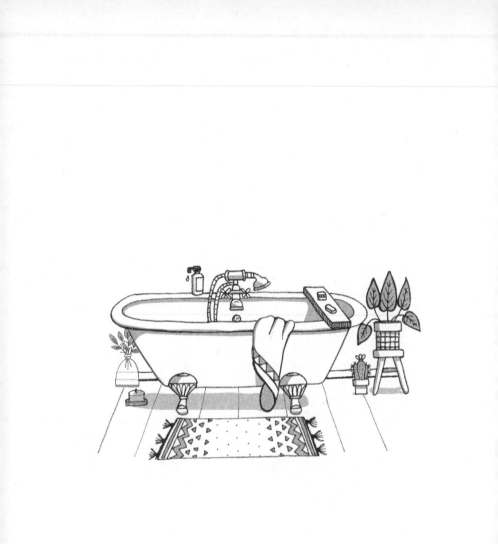

Introduction

Lights out ... and there's almost nothing nicer after a long, demanding day than nestling down under the covers in a comfy bed and drifting off to dreamland.

If only it were that easy, right?

While for some lucky people, sleep comes pretty soon after their heads hit the pillow, for others, going to bed then struggling to nod off for hours on end can become a nightmare. Especially if it's happening night after night.

If you're reading this book, you're probably having trouble sleeping. I feel for you. There's nothing nice about lying there, thoughts and worries flooding your mind, or feeling wide awake, wired and irritable, tossing and turning and simply unable to slip into slumber.

But while in the dark morning hours it can often feel like you're the only person in the world who's not fast asleep, I can tell you that you're certainly *not* alone. Research has found that in today's fast-paced, high-alert, nonstop culture almost a third of us get poor sleep most nights. Nearly three-quarters of us snooze less than the optimum seven or eight hours, and 12 percent get less than five. And lack of sleep can become a wearing long-term predicament if it's not addressed. Figures show that 35 percent of us have suffered from sleep problems for more than five years, and a fifth for more than ten. That's a lot of long, sleepless nights.

Insomnia can wreak havoc on our daytimes, too, leaving us feeling exhausted, irritable, and unwell. What's more, it has been linked to a whole host of long-term chronic conditions including type 2 diabetes, heart disease, a propensity to strokes, high blood pressure, obesity, and depression.

Yet it's not all doom and gloom. There are plenty of positive things you can do to improve your sleep. So I've trawled through the science of slumber to bring you a huge selection of assorted tricks and tips to put your body and mind in the best state possible for drifting off peacefully when you head to bed. You may be surprised to learn that everything from having a purpose in life to warming your feet, from what you eat to how you breathe, from how much time you spend outdoors to reframing your thoughts and mindset, can all help get you to sleep.

The book is packed with plenty of everyday tricks to try, as well as some weird and wonderful tips—garnered from expert research—that you can take inspiration from. What works for some might not be successful for others, so be prepared to try them out and experiment!

Sleeping well can help change your life for the better. You'll feel more energetic, optimistic, happier, and healthier when you've ditched the bad old habits that for too long have stopped you from nodding off. Remember, everyone can sleep. It's just a matter of finding out what works best for you to lure you into a long, peaceful slumber. The tips in this book will help you fall in love with falling asleep again—with little effort, no stress, and a free mind.

I hope you find the magic to help you enjoy peaceful, sleepful nights thanks to some of these sleep tricks.

Sweet dreams.

One

Before-Bed Wind-Down Tips

You can't expect your body or your mind to switch off and transition from full-on, fast, and frantic to fully relaxed and fast asleep in seconds. You need to give yourself a window in the evening in which to gradually unwind and ease yourself into peaceful tranquility. These stratagems will help steer you from tense and edgy to calm and composed, so when you lie down you've left the tensions of the day behind you and are already feeling laid back. All of which will make it easier to drift off to dreamland.

1 ✦ Turn off tech's blue light

Any type of bright light will hinder the production of the sleep hormone melatonin. But blue light—the type that's around us outside during the daytime and that is emitted from devices such as your phone, computer screen, and tablet—suppresses production the most. In a recent study published in *Chronobiology International,* researchers from the University of Haifa together with a sleep clinic exposed participants to computer screens that emitted either blue or red light from 9:00 to 11:00 PM, the hours when the pineal gland begins to produce melatonin, to see how this would affect them at bedtime.[1]

Those who were exposed to blue light produced less melatonin, slept for less time, and had more disturbed sleep. It was also found that the blue light stopped the body from activating its natural temperature-reducing mechanism—something that happens every night as a signal that it's time to sleep—and instead maintained a normal temperature throughout the night. After being exposed to red light, however, the body behaved naturally, producing melatonin and reducing its core temperature, leading to better, longer sleep.

The message? Blue light can seriously mess up your *z*'s. So stop using your electronics two to three hours before bed or use the "night shift" setting on your screens, which emits a yellowish or red light.

2 ✦ Stop being "social" before lights-out

Ignore Instagram, switch off Snapchat, turn off Twitter, and forgo Facebook well before bedtime. There's plenty of research linking social media use before bed with poor sleep.[2] Why? Because it can drive feelings of inadequacy and anxiety as we compare our lives with what's going on online—and this sort of mental angst is not conducive to dropping off without a care in the world.

When the Royal Society for Public Health published a report on how social media affects young people's health and well-being it found that Instagram and Snapchat (both image-focused) came out worst, having negative effects on sleep and body perception and inducing anxiety and a fear of missing out.[3] (Instagramxiety, anyone?) When you're scrolling social media sites, the key is to remember that people usually only post pictures where they look good and are having fun—or even snaps that are photoshopped to look perfect.

The best thing you can do is simply switch off from social media, digitally detox at least a couple of hours before bedtime, and set aside your FOMO to find your own peace—and peace of mind—so you can more easily relax into a sleep-ready state.

And while you're at it you could try embracing the Japanese concept of wabi-sabi, which shuns the shallow striving for Instagram and Pinterest perfection and instead embraces imperfection and sees beauty in cracks and flaws—including any wrinkles you may have, your less than honed and toned physique, and your lived-in home that's nurtured your family for years. There's more to life . . .

3 ✦ Rock yourself to sleep

We all know that babies find it soothing to be rocked to sleep, and it seems we're never too old to find being swayed back and forth relaxing. Researchers from the University of Geneva made the interesting discovery that adults who took a nap in a rocking bed (much like a hammock) fell asleep faster and showed an increase in the type of brain-wave activity associated with deep, restful sleep when the bed rocked than when they slept in the bed when it was stationary.[4] This suggests that a rocking motion actually helps synchronize brain wave activity into a pattern associated with sleep.

If you don't have a hammock to sleep in (and who has?), and as we're still waiting for rocking beds to become commercially available, you may want to invest in a rocking chair for the bedroom, to help lull you to sleep. So you'll look like Little Red Riding Hood's granny . . . but who cares if it gets you to sleep, right?!

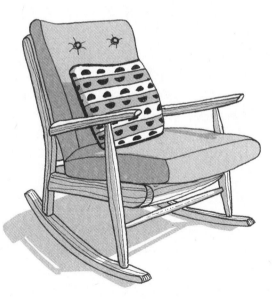

4 ✦ Do the double void

If the urge to go to the bathroom in the night often wakes you and plays havoc with your sleep, then—as well as avoiding fluids from about two hours before bed—try this trick. When getting ready for bed go pee, but after you've finished stay there for thirty seconds, then try to go again. Or go to the bathroom, say, just before cleaning your teeth, then try again after you're undressed, washed, and about to get into bed (about ten minutes later).

The technique—called double-voiding—is used to treat overactive bladder, to ensure that it's completely empty. And it could mean you get fewer rude nighttime awakenings!

5 ✦ Take a bath ninety minutes before bed

Why? Surprisingly it's not the warmth and coziness of the hot water that make you sleep, though that's undoubtedly relaxing. It all has to do with the drop in your body temperature after you get out of the bath.

Every night, your body's core temperature needs to fall to induce your brain to pump out the hormone melatonin, triggering sleepiness. When you're soaking in warm water, blood is coming to the surface of your skin—and when you get out of the bath, those dilated blood vessels rapidly radiate heat from your body's core, helping your temperature to drop quickly and sending that message to your brain to produce melatonin. A Loughborough University study found that people who took warm baths at 9:00 PM nodded off more quickly and enjoyed more slow-wave, deep sleep than those who took baths earlier in the day.[5]

6 ✦ Wash your hands

No time for a bath or shower before bed? No problem. Washing your hands with warm or cool water can have the same effect. Glabrous (nonhairy) parts of the body, such as the palms of your hands, are great at radiating heat. Though relatively small in area compared to other parts, they contain lots of special vascular structures that help you lose heat.

After washing your hands, lightly pat the skin without drying it completely; as the water evaporates, heat is dissipated from the skin's surface, thereby helping to cool your body core.

7 ✦ Ditch the dishwasher

People who are lucky enough to get a perfect night's sleep, night after night (no less), tend to have one thing in common: they stop working and have a chore curfew at least two hours before bedtime. But if there's one task you absolutely have to leave until later, then instead of rushing to stack your plates in the dishwasher after dinner, wash them by hand. Washing dishes in the sink can calm the mind and decrease stress, according to a study by Florida State University.[6] But you have to do it "mindfully"—taking time to focus on smelling the detergent and feeling the water temperature on your skin.

People who washed dishes in this way reported a 27 percent drop in anxiety. So feel free to crack open the kitchen bubbly—the dish soap, that is—before bed!

8 ✦ Don't go to bed in an argument

We've all heard this bit of advice. But now it's been proved that if you want a good night's sleep, you need to be on good terms with your other half.

A study published in the journal *Social Psychological and Personality Science* found that people who felt secure in their relationships experienced less anxiety at bedtime, which led to better quality of sleep.[7] The authors explained that restorative sleep (the high-quality, uninterrupted sleep that's healing and great for your health) only happens when you feel secure and unthreatened.

When we're children, we gain this sense of security and safeness from our parents, and when we're older the role falls to our partners. Hence, the more cared for and understood we feel, the better we sleep. So, if you've had a fight, make sure you kiss and make up before bedtime.

9 ✦ Before lights-out, lose yourself in a book

Reading is one of the best and fastest methods to de-stress you at bedtime. In one study people were given stressful tasks and then told to do one relaxing activity: reading, listening to music, having a hot drink, or playing a video game. When the stress hormone cortisol in each individual's blood was measured, it was discovered that the readers' levels had dropped the most—by 68 percent.[8] And it was a pretty quick fix, too—it took just six minutes immersed in a book to lower their heart rates and ease muscle tension.

It doesn't matter what type of book you choose—though I would advise against horror, obviously—as long as it captures your imagination and distracts you from any worries that might otherwise stop you from nodding off.

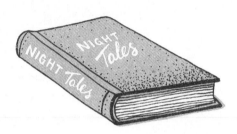

10 ✦ Set your alarm—for sleep!

Just as you set your alarm to wake you up in the morning, it's a good idea to set it in the evening to remind you it's time to start a "dimming down" routine.

You can't expect your body or your mind to simply switch off if you've been rushing around or mentally busy just before bedtime. The alarm will help prompt you to make the transition from the daytime activities that keep your brain and body buzzing—work, Facebook, exercise, internet searching, or whatever it may be—to soothing nighttime activities such as reading, listening to relaxing music, and so on. Doing something calming will help slow you down and train your mind to associate restful activities with sleep.

Make sure you choose a soothing alarm tone. Set it for forty minutes to an hour before your bedtime. Try to ensure you've done all the next-day running around you need to (ironing, sorting out school lunch boxes, and so on) before the alarm goes off, so there are no last-minute worries to interfere with wind-down time. As soon as you turn the alarm off, the first thing you should do is take a few deep breaths. This sends a message to your brain that it's time to slow down and relax.

11 ✦ Give yourself a face massage

If you're applying a moisturizer at night, then make a meal of it and give yourself a full-on facial massage.

A study published in *Complementary Therapies in Clinical Practice* found that women who had a twenty-minute facial massage experienced a drop in systolic blood pressure as well as increased feelings of sleepiness.[9]

So, start by applying pressure between your eyebrows, then slide your fingers upward, over and across your forehead, repeating several times. Next, massage from your nose to your cheeks and ears; then from your mouth across to the jawline and finish with your neck, stroking upward from the collarbone. Bliss.

12 ✦ Fall in love with lavender

Lavender oil is known for its relaxing properties and research has even proved that it can calm you down and coax you to sleep.

A study published in the *Journal of the Medical Association of Thailand* found that inhaling lavender oil reduced blood pressure and heart rate.[10] A further study, from the University of Southampton, showed that people whose rooms had been scented with lavender oil rated the quality of their sleep on average 20 percent better than those who slept in a room scented with a placebo.[11]

There are lots of ways you can use lavender oil before bed to help lull you to sleep. Try:

- spritzing your pillow with a lavender spray
- lighting a lavender-oil burner before bed (then blowing out the candle at lights-out), or using a lavender diffuser
- rubbing a couple of drops of lavender oil on your wrists, neck, chest, or temples
- adding a few drops of lavender to a hot towel and laying it over your face to inhale
- using a relaxing lavender bath oil or tying a fresh sprig of lavender to your shower head. The hot water from the shower will release the plant's essential oils.

13 ✦ Dim the lights *hygge*-style

Danes are known for their hygge lifestyle—creating coziness and contentment in their living spaces—and it could go some way to explaining why they always feature high up on the World Happiness Report. Creating hygge in your own home could improve your sleep, too.

How? Part of the way Danes create a comforting and restful atmosphere is by clever use of warm and soothing lighting from candles and low lamps (no bright overhead lights allowed!). Too much exposure to electric light at night stimulates feelings of alertness and stops the natural rise in melatonin production that darkness brings. So, if you do as the Danes do and keep the lights low in your home as the evening progresses, it will send a signal to your brain and body that it's time to rest.

Try dining by candlelight, use the dimmer switch on your overhead lights, or—better still—use lamps with low-wattage, dimmable bulbs.

14 ✦ And keep the lights low

So, you've dimmed the lights downstairs to prompt your melatonin levels to rise nicely in preparation for sleep. But make sure you don't ruin the effect when you go upstairs by switching on bright lights in the bathroom while brushing your teeth (and in your bedroom while reading a book). An Australian study revealed that just one hour of bright light was enough to reduce nighttime production of melatonin to almost daytime quantities.[12]

Use low-lit bedside lamps and, if your bathroom lights are dim-mable, look at installing a dimmer switch.

15 ✦ Curb binge-watching

Lots of us can't resist the urge to watch "just one more" episode before bed. But binge-watching—the relatively new phenomenon of guzzling episode after episode of a gripping TV series in quick succession—could be stopping us from getting a decent night's kip. A US and Belgian study published in the *Journal of Clinical Sleep Medicine* found that serious binge-viewing habits were associated with poor sleep, fatigue, and symptoms of insomnia, whereas regular television viewing wasn't.[13] It's thought that the increased mental stimulation linked to the watchers' high degree of engagement with such television shows leads to so much pre-sleep arousal that it interferes with the ability to drift off.

Set yourself a strict limit as to how many episodes you watch a night and take a break after each one to rid yourself of the automatic urge to keep on watching.

16 ✦ Legs up the wall

Ask any yoga teacher to suggest poses that might possibly persuade you to fall asleep and the chances are *viparita karani,* or legs-up-the-wall, will be high up the list. This posture is thought to trigger the parasympathetic nervous system, helping to slow the heart rate and encourage relaxation. It's simple to do and doesn't require too much flexibility.

Start by sitting on the floor with one hip, left or right, against the wall. Then turn your body and, keeping your buttocks close to the wall, bring your legs up onto it while gently lowering your back to the floor. Use a pillow next to the wall or under your hips or lower back to help support you if necessary, and get comfortably into position—nearer or further away from the wall as best suits you, and slightly bending your knees if you need to.

Stay in the position for a few minutes or for as long as you feel comfortable. You can do this in bed with your legs up against the headboard, if that's practical.

17 ✦ Go into child's pose

This is another popular yoga pose that can relax both body and mind as well as ease tension in the lower back. You can do this one in bed or on the floor.

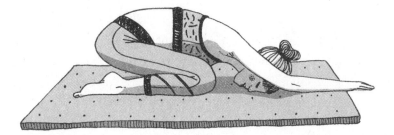

First get into a kneeling position, sitting on your heels, with knees together or hip-distance apart, whichever feels more comfortable.

Next, roll the top half of your body forward until your forehead rests on the bed or floor with arms outstretched in front of you. You can rest your head on a pillow if it's too much of a strain'to come all the way forward.

Hold the pose for as long as comfortable and for a maximum of three minutes, breathing slowly.

18 ✦ Dangle like a rag doll

Stretches like this one, which require no strength and little balance, can calm your mind, release tension, and help you wind down for sleep.

- ✦ Standing with your arms raised overhead, begin to fold forward from your hips, reaching down toward your toes, then hang there like a rag doll.
- ✦ Allow all your muscles and your head to hang heavy and feel the tension release from your shoulders. Loosely shake your arms back and forth and soften your knees as much as necessary for your own comfort.
- ✦ Dangle for as long as you feel comfortable, closing your eyes, breathing slowly, and letting your thoughts drift.
- ✦ While you're there, try sighing every time you breathe out. Research shows that the act of sighing can actually relieve stress and muscle tension.[14] Ahhhhh.

19 ✦ Listen to soothing music

In a study published in the *Journal of Advanced Nursing* students who listened to relaxing classical music for forty-five minutes at bed-time over three weeks fell asleep sooner, slept better and for longer, and experienced fewer depressive symptoms than those who didn't.[15]

If you enjoy lying back and listening to some tranquil beats to help you sleep, search out music that's string-based, with no extreme variations in volume and no repeated melody. This allows your mind to wander dreamily because you're not anticipating the repeat. Ideally, the music should have around 50 to 70 beats per minute—the theory is that your heartbeat slows to synchronize with the rhythm.

20 ✦ Feel all tingly

Who knew that listening to someone whisper while they brush their hair could set off your autonomous sensory meridian response (ASMR) and send you to sleep?

Let me explain. ASMR describes a tingling, calming, and relaxing sensation that starts at the top of your head and spreads to the neck, spine, and shoulders and sometimes the arms and legs, too. It's the feeling you may get when being massaged, for example.

Visual and audio ASMR clips—designed to induce this tingling sensation—are springing up all over the Internet and especially on YouTube. They feature simple, repetitive, slow, gentle, or crisp sounds such as rain falling, whispering, tapping, or scratching, or even someone doing calming things such as folding freshly washed towels, flicking through a magazine, or brushing their hair.

One study by researchers at Swansea University found that 82 percent of people who listened to ASMR clips did it to help them sleep, and 98 percent to help them relax.[16] A new study by Sheffield University found that people watching these videos experienced a reduction in heart rate of 3.14 beats a minute.[17]

So listening to whispering really may be good for your health. It's certainly a different way to help you get to sleep. And if it's watching people fold their laundry that lulls you to the Land of Nod, then why not?!

21 ✦ A stroll at sundown?

A Japanese study found that a forest walk improved the slumber of people who usually had difficulty sleeping.[18] They dropped off sooner, and slept better and for longer. Furthermore, a late afternoon walk was more successful in this respect than taking a walk earlier in the day.

This may be to do with the fact that when we're outdoors and exposed to the natural light of dusk, it helps synchronize our body clocks, making us feel sleepy as darkness falls.

So don't sit inside under electric light and deprive yourself of outdoor darkness—go for a leisurely walk when the light is fading.

22 ✦ Write a detailed to-do list

Get out a paper and pen before lights-out and jot down what needs doing over the next few days.

Writing a to-do list at bedtime can help you fall asleep faster. A study published in the *Journal of Experimental Psychology* monitored the sleep of two groups.[19] The first was asked to spend five minutes drawing up a list of things they needed to remember to do in the next few days. The other half had to write down tasks they'd completed in the last few days.

Interestingly, the group who wrote the to-do lists fell asleep within about fifteen minutes whereas the other group took an average of twenty-five. And the more detailed and specific the person's list was, the quicker he or she fell asleep.

The researchers surmised that "off-loading" on paper the things that have to be done, and the actual act of writing them all down, helps free the mind from responsibility and stops that list from going round and round in your mind as you try to sleep.

So make a list—and be specific and thorough.

23 ✦ Fold forward

This is a nice easy stretch you can do while sitting on the edge of the bed that can prepare you for sleep.

Simply sit, then fold forward at the hips, letting your head and arms dangle gently, and placing your fingers lightly around your ankles to help anchor yourself. Breathing slowly and deeply, stay like this for up to sixty seconds—if at any point it feels uncomfortable, slowly rise out of the position.

In yoga, any head-below-heart pose, or inversion, such as this one is thought to calm and relax the nervous system.

24 ✦ Rock on your feet

Rocking is known to be relaxing and to promote sleepiness, and if you rock on your feet the movement can also release stress and tension by stimulating acupressure points in the feet.

Try this before you get into bed:

- ✦ Stand straight with your feet shoulder width apart. Now shift your body weight onto your heels, so that your toes lift off the floor.
- ✦ Next, shift your weight onto your toes so that your heels rock off the floor.
- ✦ Continue rocking back and forth slowly and smoothly for a few minutes, breathing deeply as you do so, then get into bed.

25 ✦ Grow roots and feel grounded

You can do this exercise after the previous one ("Rock on your feet") or on its own. It's simple, but very effective at helping your body relax and your mind feel grounded and free of stress and worries.

Stand on the spot, feet shoulder width apart, and breathe smoothly and deeply. Imagine yourself feeling heavier and try to sink all that weight into your feet, grounding them in the floor.

Now, as you sink into the floor, imagine your feet growing roots that keep you stable. Stay in this position for a few minutes, if you feel comfortable. It will not only ground you physically, but mentally, too—and help transfer stress and energy from your mind into the floor beneath you.

If you find the exercise difficult, sometimes covering the crown of your head with your hands can help.

26 ✦ Take a tai chi shower

This technique helps you metaphorically wash away stress and tension from your mind and body before bed.

First, either sit or kneel in a comfortable position. Then, imagine you are seated in a warm pool underneath a shower or waterfall. Feel the warm water trickle steadily over your head and body, or feel it gush over you, whichever you find more pleasant.

Revel and relax in the feeling of being bathed by warm, fragrant water. As it flows, imagine it washing away all your stress, too. Envision your tension leaving you as bubbles are carried away downstream.

27 ✦ Have a cup of chamomile

Don't like cocoa before bed? Try a cup of chamomile instead.

Chamomile tea has long been known for its soothing properties. In an Iranian study, nursing-home residents with sleep troubles were given either 200 mg of chamomile extract twice daily, or a placebo.[20] Those who took the chamomile showed a significant improvement in their sleep. Another, Taiwanese, study showed that postnatal women with sleep problems who drank chamomile tea for two weeks slept better and experienced fewer symptoms of depression.[21]

It's thought that the flavonoid apigenin in the flowerheads of the chamomile plant may have a sedative effect because it acts on benzodiazepine receptors in the brain.

You can buy chamomile as teabags or as loose tea flowers. Brew for two to five minutes, depending on your strength preference.

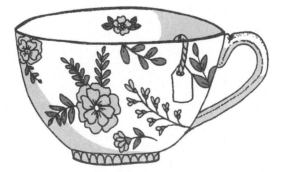

28 ✦ Warm your eyes and the back of your neck before bed

If you've ever had a facial or neck massage using warm oils, you'll know the blissful sense of comfort, contentment, and relaxation it can induce. A recent Japanese study found that warming both these regions of the body to around 104 degrees Fahrenheit (40 degrees Celsius) before bed can help you fall asleep better and get more deep sleep, too.[22]

The researchers asked volunteers with mild sleeping difficulties to try three experiments for five days each: for ten minutes before bedtime, warming the skin around the eyes, using a special device; for thirty minutes before bedtime, warming the skin at the back of the neck; and as a control, no treatment at all.

The results? Both warming the eyes and warming the neck led to better, deeper sleep. Heating these areas helps reduce sympathetic-nervous activity and increase parasympathetic-nervous activity, which helps slow heart rate and encourages relaxation.

You can buy "warming" eye masks and microwavable (heatable) neck pillows if you'd like to give this trick a try.

29 ✦ Hug your knees — and rock 'n' roll

The knees-toward-chest pose in yoga helps release tension in the body. You can do this move on the floor before getting into bed or when you're actually in bed.

Lying down, draw your knees up to your chest and hug them gently toward your body. Feel the tension in your lower back ease and enjoy the feeling of comfort as you hold your knees against you.

Hugging—even if you are doing it to yourself—releases the hormone oxytocin, the "love hormone," which is thought to reduce your stress response as well as any anxiety you may be experiencing. Not only that, but just being in this fetal position can have a calming and comforting effect on the mind, and it helps gently massage your lower back.

Breathe deeply as you hug your knees and, if it feels comfortable to do so, rock gently and slowly from side to side (this helps to massage your spine). You can synchronize your breathing to your rocking— inhale as you roll to the left, exhale as you come to the center, inhale as you roll to the right, exhale back to the center. Or rock and breathe in whichever way relaxes you best. A study published in the journal *Current Biology* found that by boosting sleep-related brain waves the rocking motion led to more deep sleep.[23]

After a while you may feel too dozy to continue rocking, so lie in the middle position, gently hugging your knees and taking a few more breaths before slowly lowering them back to the floor or bed.

30 ✦ Do a pre-bed meditation

It has been found that people who meditate enjoy better-quality, deeper sleep than those who don't.[24] This could be due to the fact that—remarkably—regular meditation appears to have the capacity to change the structure of your brain as well as help you feel less stressed.

A Harvard-affiliated team at Massachusetts General Hospital took magnetic resonance (MR) brain images of a group of people before and after they took part in an eight-week mindfulness program, meditating for an average of twenty-seven minutes a day. Results showed an increase in grey-matter density in areas of the brain associated with empathy and the regulation of emotions, and a diminished concentration of grey matter in the amygdala, an area associated with anxiety and stress.[25] What's more, it has also been found that meditating before bed can significantly increase our output of melatonin, the sleep-inducing hormone.[26]

Spend time before lights-out winding down with a few moments of meditation. Sit cross-legged on the floor or on the bed, or do it lying down in bed, whichever you prefer. You can follow guided meditations on a podcast or with apps such as Headspace or Calm.

A simple wind-down you could try tonight is the "100 steps" meditation. First, imagine you are at the top of a gently sloping hill. Perhaps it's a perfect summer's afternoon. A warm sun is shining; flowers, their faces toward the sun, are visited by humming bees and butterflies. Starting at 100, begin to make your way down the hill, counting down and exhaling with each step you take.

Let your breath come naturally—don't try to breathe faster or slower, more deeply or shallowly, than is comfortable and calming. If your mind wanders, don't worry. Just tell yourself "I got distracted" and continue with the counting and the breathing.

31 ✦ Stare at something

Another easy introduction to meditation is *trataka,* or "yogic gazing." It involves fixing your eyes on an object (usually a candle flame) and completely focusing on it. Yoga experts say that doing this can help clear your mind to help you sleep. It also flexes your concentration muscle, so the more you practice it the easier it is to meditate.

First, light a candle a few feet away and directly in front of you, and sit comfortably so that the flame is almost level with your eyes. Make sure there are no drafts, so that the flame remains steady. Breathing regularly, gaze at the flame without blinking, for as long as is comfortable. As thoughts enter your mind, be aware of them, then let them go, trying to keep your focus on the flame.

When your eyes start to water and you need to blink, close them and you'll see an after-image of the flame on the inside of your lids. Try to steady the image at the point of your third eye in between your eyebrows. When the image fades, begin gazing at the flame again.

If you don't like the feeling of staring at a flame—or can't be sure you'll remember to blow out the candle before bed—you can choose to focus on anything you like: say, a picture of a flower or a tree. Alternatively, there are plenty of online videos featuring candles that you can use.

32 + Feel the love

Loving-kindness meditation is a practice that's designed to boost feelings of compassion—both for yourself and for others. And it can be a nurturing way of helping you lull yourself to sleep. A study from the University of Arizona found that just ten minutes of loving-kindness meditation had an immediate relaxing effect on those who tried it.[27] Their breathing rates dropped, and the variability of their heart rates increased, indicating relaxation.

The practice has been linked with everything from easing pain, depression, and post-traumatic stress disorder to promoting general well-being, as well as making people more sociable and positive in their emotions. Phew! Can you afford *not* to give this a try?

Here's how to do it yourself, before or after lights-out:

Lie back and breathe deeply and slowly.

Place one or both hands on your heart. Imagine feeling completely at ease, surrounded by compassion, breathing out your anxiety and breathing in peace, calm, and love.

Mentally repeat some phrases of love and kindness toward your-self, things like:

+ May I be happy.
+ May I be well.
+ May I be peaceful.
+ May I be free from pain.
+ May I be free from anxiety.

Let all these feelings wrap you in a safe, warm cocoon of calm and ease for a few moments.

Next, direct those feelings onto someone you love or you're close to—your partner, child, parents, sibling, friend:

- May you be happy.
- May you be well.
- May you be peaceful.
- May you be free from suffering . . .

and so on.

You can then, if you want to, extend the feelings to other people in your life: to acquaintances you may not know that well, or generally to people around the world who may be facing conflict or hardship, or even to someone you feel resentment or anger toward (although this can take some application!).

Do what feels comfortable. Keep the meditation simple by focusing on yourself and others close to you, if that's easier—or expand it as far as you feel happy to do.

The important thing is to experience a sense of peaceful loving-kindness. This may help you nod off tranquilly; or you can use the practice any time you feel in need of a pick-me-up or calm-me-down.

33 ✦ Lift up the sky

Qigong (pronounced "chee-gung") is an ancient Chinese health practice combining gentle, fluid stretching movements with mental concentration and breathing.

A study published in the *Journal of Health Psychology* found that people who participated in qigong sessions for thirty minutes, three times a week, slept longer and reported enhanced psychological well-being compared with people who hadn't practiced the discipline.[28]

A simple qigong movement to try before bed that can calm your mind and release stress in your body is called "lifting the sky."

✦ First stand with your feet hip-width apart.

✦ With your palms facing the floor, point your fingers toward each other, leaving a small space and keeping your arms as straight as is comfortable. Tilt your neck downward to look at your hands.

✦ Next, with your head following the movement of your hands, lift them up in front of you and above your head in an arc movement.

✦ When your hands reach the top of the arc, gently push them up as if lifting the sky, stretching your spine as you do so.

✦ Then lower your arms as if you're a bird flapping its wings, and bring them to your sides, breathing out with an open-mouthed "ahhh" sound.

✦ Repeat four times.

You can do a version of this exercise while lying in bed, too—though only if there's no one next to you, or you're liable to give them an unwelcome whack!

And why not join a class, or copy movements from online videos?

34 ✦ Listen to a bedtime story

If you were read bedtime stories as a child, you'll know how easily they can soothe and send you to the Land of Nod. Well, just because you're now an adult, it doesn't mean you can't get lulled to sleep with a tale or two. And while it might be a little weird to ask your parents to read to you when you're over eighteen, there are plenty of apps and audiobooks that can step up to the mark.

For example, the popular Calm app has a section of sleep stories especially recorded for adults, featuring the dulcet tones of actors including Stephen Fry. They obviously hit the mark, because within eighteen months of launching, the stories had been listened to over sixty-three million times.

You could also sign up to Audible, the online audiobook giant. Search online for suitable podcasts or listen to CDs of your favorite childhood story (think *Wind in the Willows* or *The Jungle Book*).

Choose your easy-listening wisely. Don't opt for crime or thrillers at bedtime—go for something that's not too exciting or gripping, or you'll take ages to drift off to dreamland. The plot has to be interesting enough to distract you from any worries without being so complicated you have to concentrate hard.

You might want to buy a pillow speaker that plugs into your audio device and tucks under your pillow so you don't disturb your partner with your nighttime listening.

35 ✦ Stretch the day's stresses away

Stretching helps you relax by loosening any tension you're holding in your body, which is particularly important if you spend all day sitting at a desk. One study published in the journal *Sleep* found that women who embarked on a year-long session of stretching exercises reported better sleep.[29] Other studies have found that stretching your legs before bed can relieve symptoms of both restless legs syndrome and leg cramps—both common conditions that interfere with getting to, and staying, asleep.[30]

Try this set of evening stretches to help you wind down for sleep. Hold all the stretches for four or five breaths. Stop if you feel any pain, and don't overstretch. All your moves should be done slowly and without straining. Don't worry if you can't seem to stretch very far—that will come with time.

◆ Kneel on the floor and raise both your arms above your head, looking upward as you do so, leaning slightly backward and opening up your chest.

◆ Now bend forward, reaching your arms out in front of you, lowering your forehead as close to the floor as you can, and keeping your bottom on your heels.

✦ Go onto all fours, straighten your arms and legs, and raise your hips and buttocks into the air, looking toward your knees.

✦ In bed, try the butterfly stretch. Lying on your back, place the soles of your feet together and let your knees gently lower to either side of you. Place pillows beneath your knees if that feels more comfortable. You'll feel your hips, inner thighs, and back stretch. Be careful not to overstretch. Breathe slowly and deeply. You may even find you drop off in this position.

36 ✦ Say "om"

If you've ever been to a yoga class, you may have begun and ended your session with an "om." This chanting practice is thought to have spiritual powers that help connect you to the universe. And on a simpler level? Saying om before bedtime could help you get to sleep!

Chanting has been shown to calm your bodily responses. In one survey women with high blood pressure were instructed to chant om for five minutes, and in so doing they both experienced an immediate drop in blood pressure and reduced their heart rate by six beats a minute, indicating a state of calm.[31] Another study used functional magnetic resonance imaging (fMRI) to measure brain activity in the participants, who were asked to chant either "om" or "sss."[32]

The outcome? The om group showed deactivation in areas of the limbic brain—including the amygdala, which is associated with emotional responses such as anxiety. There were no changes in the sss group. It's thought that the vibration sensation of om stimulates the vagus nerve, which helps switch on our parasympathetic nervous system, responsible for the calming response.

Try sitting upright in bed, breathe in slowly and deeply, then on the exhale say "om" until you have no breath left.

There's a right way to say it, by the way. It should sound like the letter *o* drawn out and the sound *mmm*—like "home" with the *h* dropped.

Namaste!

Two

Mind Tricks

To nod off, you need a quiet, peaceful mind—one that's not filled with worries about what happened during the day, what might happen tomorrow, or how long you're going to be lying there tossing and turning.

Often, the only time we have complete peace and quiet is when our heads hit the pillow or if we wake in the middle of the night. But the trouble is, that quiet—with no distractions—is pretty much the perfect opportunity for our so-called monkey mind to chatter at us incessantly and be heard loud and clear, filling our thoughts with to-do and not-to-do lists, anxieties and apprehensions, worst-case scenarios and what-ifs, ruminations and deliberations.... Exhausting! And if your busy brain won't switch off, you won't nod off either.

Fighting against anxious thoughts will only make them loom larger, so try these tricks to help calm and distract your mind, or take it off to a better, stiller, and more serene and soothing place—perfect for drifting off to dreamland.

37 ✦ Think of five good things

Forget about counting sheep. Count yourself lucky. Every night, write down or say aloud five things that were good about your day. They can be as simple as getting a cup of tea made for you in the office or bagging a bargain in the supermarket. Expert psychological studies carried out by UK and Canadian universities have demonstrated that writing a gratitude journal, or just thinking about what's good in your life at bedtime rather than what's bad, can help you fall asleep faster and for longer.[1] So go on—for a sounder sleep, try cultivating an attitude of gratitude.

38 ✦ Speak—don't think

If your mind is a whirlwind of worry when you hit the sack, try speaking! Talking out loud engages parts of the brain different from those responsible for internal negative ruminations. It also helps slow things down—our thoughts can race much faster than we can physically speak. You could simply say something like "Slow down" every time worries enter your head, then speak positive thoughts or possible solutions to combat the concern you're fretting over.

One study carried out by Bangor University gave participants a set of written instructions, and asked them to read them either silently or out loud.[2] Concentration and performance were measured, and both were better in those who had read out the instructions. Hearing yourself seems to help you gain more control of a situation.

So, if you're anxious about a large unexpected bill that's come in, for example, try saying out loud: "I just need to look over the bank statement tomorrow and start writing out a budget for the month. It can easily be paid if we're a little more careful for the next couple of weeks."

This tactic works just as well if you whisper, by the way. Waking your partner at night by loudly declaiming will not be conducive to a restful sleep for either of you!

39 ✦ The elephant in the bedroom

If you were told not to think about a white elephant before going to bed, the chances are that a white elephant would keep popping up in your thoughts quite a lot. Likewise, trying to suppress a worrying thought at bedtime can often have the reverse effect—and stress you out in the process.

In one interesting study, researchers from the University of Oxford asked their volunteers to select a thought most likely to dominate their pre-sleep; it could be anything from a concern about finances to not being able to drop off. They were then split into two groups: the first group were told to try to suppress the particular thought, and the second to simply relax and let their thoughts come and go. Guess what? The first group took longer to fall asleep and their sleep was more disturbed than the second, free-thinking group's.[3]

Actively, or aggressively, telling yourself to suppress a thought can not only make it loom larger, but it can also agitate your brain, putting it into busy task mode ("Don't think about x or y!") rather than "relax" mode (zzzzz). So try to let your thoughts come and go at bedtime without trying to get rid of them—but at the same time without dwelling on them.

Acknowledge a worrying thought and tell it, calmly, "Thank you for popping into my mind. I can't do anything about you at the moment, so I'll deal with you tomorrow." Keeping a tranquil mind tells your brain you're not on high alert about anything; it doesn't need to do anything just now toward solving a problem—thus, you are far more likely to fall asleep.

40 ✦ Try to stay awake

Sounds crazy, but it might just work. Researchers asked one group of insomniacs to attempt to fall asleep as they normally would, and another group to lie in bed, keep their eyes open, and try to stay awake for as long as possible. Result? The second group fell asleep faster—and reported less anxiety about drifting off.[4]

It is because sleep is an automatic process, the researchers surmised, that trying to fall asleep can actually inhibit the process. Plus, going to bed without the pressure of *having to* fall asleep also seems to help.

41 ✦ Send your mind off to a happy place

A golden-sanded beach, a shady riverside walk, a crystal-clear water-fall, or a field of colorful wild flowers.... Researchers at the University of Oxford found that insomniacs who were told to visualize a "happy place" or a relaxing scene drifted off to sleep twenty minutes sooner than when instructed to think of nothing or to count sheep.[5]

It was surmised that counting sheep was simply too tedious to distract the insomniacs from any worries they were having, whereas using imagery to immerse themselves in a happy place was engrossing enough to distract them. Further research has shown that, compared to good sleepers, insomniacs tend to summon up fewer images but experience a higher percentage of unpleasant ones when they try to sleep.[6]

So conjuring up a pleasant view might just do it for you.

42 ✦ Use your five senses

When you are visualizing your happy place make it as vivid as possible by using your five senses. What do you see, hear, taste, touch, and smell?

As well as seeing the idyllic scenery in your mind's eye, hear the distant noise of seagulls overhead, the gentle lapping of waves; feel the heat on your face, the soft sand between your toes; breathe in the smell of the salty air and imagine the taste of a cooling cocktail.

Using all five senses helps to keep you zoned away from any unwanted thoughts, really immersing you in and engaging with your "happy place."

43 ✦ Pen and paper by the bed

Ever woken up and suddenly remembered a bill you haven't paid, a note you've forgotten to send in to school, or someone's birthday? Or maybe these thoughts pop into your head at bedtime? They're not exactly world problems that you need to dwell on, but they'll probably keep you awake because your brain is concerned that you might forget what you've just remembered by morning time. Keep pen and paper by the bed so you can jot down all these reminders. That way, you're giving your brain permission to forget about them for the night—so you can nod off.

44 ✦ Play mind games

Give your brain a mental exercise to do when you hit the hay. A study from Southern Illinois University found that giving insomniacs moderately difficult mental arithmetic problems to do at bedtime made them fall asleep faster.[7]

Try counting backward from 100—or even 1,000—in groups of 5. If you want to make it more difficult and ensure your mind doesn't wander, count back in groups of 4, 7, 12, or 18, for example. Concentrating on a mental task like this helps focus away from any worries. Also, just the rhythmic pattern of counting in blocks could help lull you to sleep.

If math just isn't your thing, try other mind games: think of cities beginning with A, animals beginning with B, and so on.

One thing to note, though: the study found that people who didn't have sleep problems took *longer* to get to sleep playing these games. So only use this trick on nights you're having trouble!

45 ✦ Sing a lullaby . . . to yourself

You may feel silly—but singing yourself a childhood lullaby that holds positive associations with sleep can trigger the same relaxed and "safe" state of mind in you now.

Focusing on the act of singing will also help filter out other things going on in your mind. Plus, the movements our mouths make when we sing encourage the jaw to loosen—good for those of us who hold tension there when we're stressed, which can stop us from unwinding enough to fall asleep.

The perfect pace of a lullaby? About 60 to 80 beats per minute, which replicates a resting heartbeat. One study by Case Western Reserve University found that people who listened to soothing music at this tempo slept better, and for longer, too.[8]

46 ✦ Chant a mantra

Do you find yourself lying in bed and berating yourself over something you did or didn't do, should or shouldn't have said, during the day?

When your mind won't let you sleep because you're beating yourself up over something, then try repeating a silent mantra. Research published in the *Brain and Behavior* journal found that repeating a word to yourself over and over can calm your mind by reducing activity in all areas of the brain, most notably the part called the "default mode network," which is responsible for self-judgment and self-reflection.[9]

Choose a word with positive connotations—something like "good," "happy," or "fine." Repeat the word over and over again in your mind, focusing on it as a mantra. If your mind wanders, bring it back to the mantra and the worrying thoughts should soon abate.

47 ✦ Shuffle images for better shut-eye

Cognitive shuffling, or serial diverse imagining, is a way of helping you fall asleep created by the cognitive scientist Dr. Luc P. Beaudoin. It's designed to distract your mind from any analytical thinking and problem solving that might be going on in your brain at bedtime and keeping you awake. It does this by encouraging you to think of a "dreamy parade of sundry images" that have no connection to each other.

Sleep research has discovered that as we fall asleep we often conjure up a range of diverse, fleeting visual images and have "micro-dreams," and that these images may actually help us drop off. And this method is intended to transport your brain to this hazy pre-sleep picture-seeing state.

Here's how to do it:

* First, think of a word of five letters or more, preferably with no recurring letters—for example, "bridge."
* Then, with the first letter of the word think up as many different images as you can. For example, "bottle"—imagine drinking a bottle of cool water; "balloon"—imagine it rising into a clear blue sky; "bluebell"—imagine a woody glade filled with bluebells.
* Continue generating words and images until you get stuck or bored, then go on to the next letter of the word.

If you find it too difficult, there's an app, mySleepButton, that leads you through the process.

48 ✦ Get out of bed?

One way of preventing sleeplessness is to build a strong association between your bed and sleep. So if you toss and turn and struggle to fall asleep or to get back to sleep after waking, many experts suggest that after fifteen or twenty minutes, you should get out of bed. It sounds counterintuitive, but the theory is that getting up will help you stop associating your bed with being awake and frustrated.

I'd put in a caveat here, though. If after those fifteen or twenty minutes you're lying in bed awake but feel relaxed and at ease, stay there. That's perfectly fine. But if you're restless, uncomfortable, and anxious, then get up. Go downstairs or sit in a chair or beanbag in your bedroom, and do something mundane such as listening to soothing music or reading a (nonthrilling) book in low light. As soon as you start to feel sleepy again, slowly get up and climb back into bed.

This all helps to reinforce in your mind that your bed is a place of sleepiness, not restlessness.

If getting out of bed feels like too big a leap, you can always try sitting up in bed, or getting out from under the covers and sitting on the side of the bed, and reading or listening to music. Then when you feel sleepy, lie down again. That way you're still reinforcing the association of lying down in bed with sleepiness.

49 ✦ Label your emotions—put your feelings into words

When, under the covers, worries flood your mind and you start to feel completely caught up in them, your amygdala—the part of the brain that's linked to your fight-or-flight response—can go into overdrive. But if you give those emotions you're feeling a label or identity by saying "I'm angry," "I'm stressed," "I'm anxious," or "I'm overwhelmed," for example, you can effectively put a stop to that emotional response.

Research from the University of California, Los Angeles, published in the journal *Psychological Science*, found that by so doing, less activity in the amygdala was recorded and more in the right ventrolateral prefrontal cortex, a part of the brain that stops you overreacting.[10] And in another study by the same university, participants who were scared of spiders and who were told to label their anxious emotions showed the least physiological signs of fear such as a racing heart.[11]

Try naming each anxious emotion as it comes into your head; you may well find it lessens the intensity of your feelings and helps your mind quiet down so you can nod off.

50 ✦ Try biofeedback

This is another therapy that aims to help you use your thoughts to control your stress responses, so it's especially good for people who struggle to relax or feel anxious at bedtime. There are therapists who can carry out the technique. It involves placing electrodes on different parts of the body, which measure your stress responses such as muscle tension and heart rate. The therapist will then teach you how to try to relax and control that response.

There are different types of biofeedback—for instance, in neurofeedback sensors are placed on the head to measure brain activity. If you're nervous and lots of concerns are flying around your mind, the sensors will pick up fast brain waves. The therapist will then help you to relax and calm your mind and the sensors will show slower, more relaxed brain waves.

In respiratory feedback, sensors are placed around the chest and abdomen to record your breathing pattern. The therapist will teach a stressed breather to breathe slowly through the abdomen. Ask your doctor or other health care professional for recommended biofeedback practitioners.

There are also home biofeedback devices, interactive computer programs, and apps you can try out for yourself.

51 ✦ Stop catastrophizing your sleeplessness

Fear and anxiety about how your sleeplessness might affect your health or your ability to cope can just make sleep issues worse. A typical scenario might go like this: You're lying in bed unable to sleep. You start to panic because you have a busy day tomorrow and you're worried you're not going to be able to manage everything. If you can't manage your workload, you'll look stupid in front of your colleagues and your boss. There's been talk of layoffs, so you may even lose your job. If you lose your job, you'll lose your house or your apartment.... The cycle of worry and anxiety worsens so there's now even less of a chance you'll fall asleep.

Cognitive behavioral therapy for insomnia (CBT-i) has been shown to be a really effective tool to help reduce the type of anxiety that many of us feel about not being able to fall asleep and stay asleep. Part of the therapy involves recognizing negative, exaggerated, and inaccurate thoughts about sleep, then breaking the cycle by challenging them as they arrive in your head and replacing them with other far more realistic ones.

So, for example, as the thought "If I don't fall asleep within ten minutes, I'll never make it through tomorrow" fills your head, try to see it for what it is: an untruth and an exaggeration. Then, try replacing it with a more realistic thought, such as "I've had sleepless nights before and I've always managed to get through the following day. I'm just going to stop worrying about falling asleep and enjoy the fact that I am lying down and relaxing; simply resting will do me good."

Regularly practicing this technique can help you change the negative exaggerated thought patterns that hype you up at night and make it harder to fall asleep. For extra help on this, try our next tip, too ("Put your thoughts on trial").

52 ✦ Put your thoughts on trial

It may be helpful to keep a thought record to help you work out whether many of your opinions about your sleeplessness are true or if they tend to magnify the negative and pounce on the worst-case scenario. Thought records push you to put your thoughts on trial as you look for the evidence for and against your thought.

You can make your own thought record in a notebook or download a template from the Internet (a simple search for "cognitive behavioral therapy thought record" will come up with results). Fill out the form every time you have a strong or upsetting thought about sleep, be it in the daytime or nighttime when you're in bed.

Typically, the form will have headings such as the following. Below each heading I've included an example of a thought you may have about sleep and the sort of comments you may give:

The thought I'm having about sleep
I'm lying in bed unable to sleep. I need eight hours tonight. Why can't I sleep?! There's something wrong with me.

How the thought makes me feel

Anxious, panicky, tearful, hopeless.

Is there a more realistic, balanced version of your thought?

It would be nice to get a solid eight hours but not everyone needs that amount of sleep to function well—there's plenty of evidence to support the belief that people can manage on much less than that. There's nothing seriously wrong with me. It's impossible to have an inability to fall asleep. I'm feeling stressed because I've taken on too much work and my mind is overactive at night. That could be interfering with my ability to relax and fall asleep. I need to cut back on work and give myself a little more me-time.

How I feel now

More optimistic, less negative, more in control.

After filling out thought records for a while, you should find it easier to recognize and challenge the unhelpful thoughts you get at bedtime, when it's often far too easy to imagine the worst. You'll come to realize that you don't have to believe every catastrophic thought you have about sleeping.

Interestingly, many people who revisit their bedtime remarks in "the thought I'm having about sleep" section during the day are shocked by the disaster scenarios they've committed to paper. Their daytime rational mind sees those thoughts as unreasonable and exaggerated.

Carrying out this exercise regularly could help you put a rein on catastrophic thinking at nighttime, as you become more able to rationalize your thoughts—even in the dark of the night.

53 ✦ Tap into better sleep

Emotional freedom technique (EFT), or "tapping," is a therapy thought to help release negative emotions like stress or anxiety. Sometimes called psychological acupuncture, it involves quickly tapping various energy pathways around the body to rewire neural pathways in the brain, helping you to see a situation in a more positive light. One Korean university study found it was a useful tool to combat insomnia in older people.[12]

You can learn the technique from a therapist or in a class, but a simple exercise you can use in bed if you're feeling stressed is to tap with two or three fingers on the "karate chop point" of your hand—the fleshy spot just below the little finger. Focus on what you feel anxious about as you tap, and it could help you change your perspective on what's worrying you and calm you to sleep.

54 ✦ Use positive bedtime affirmations

"I fall asleep so easily . . . there's nothing to it!" Using positive statements (affirmations) like this could help you change any self-sabotaging thoughts you have about sleep.

Our minds are constantly influenced by what people say to us. For example, if someone says "You look tired," you may begin to feel that way even if you felt wide awake until that moment. In the same way, we can influence our minds to approach sleep positively—to see it as something natural and attainable, and not something to worry about not getting enough of—by telling ourselves optimistic, encouraging things about it. Our brains form new neural connections all the time. By regularly repeating positive affirmations about sleep, we can create new pathways in the brain, reprogramming our minds to feel differently about it. It's called neuroplasticity: the ability of the brain to change and adapt.

There are just a couple of rules about using affirmations: they need to be in the present tense and can't contain negative words like "can't" or "won't."

Try addressing statements to yourself like the ones below as you do your nighttime routine. Look at yourself in the mirror as you say them out loud, or just run them through your mind if you don't want to look too loopy:

"I can easily fall asleep gently and peacefully."
"I like going into my bedroom. It's such a lovely place of calm and relaxation."
"I drift off to sleep easily and stay peaceful throughout the night."

Repeat the affirmations every night and several times through the day to keep convincing your mind what a superb sleeper you are.

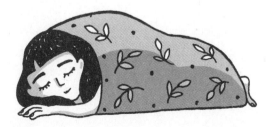

55 ✦ In bed, be in the moment

Mindfulness meditation can be a great tool to help you sleep. It involves shifting your brain away from "doing" mode (worrying, contemplating, analyzing, problem solving … all things that can stop you from sleeping) to "being" mode—simply being in the present, usually by focusing on your breathing. The aim is not to make your worrying thoughts simply stop, but rather to observe those thoughts, acknowledge them, and then allow them to pass without acting or dwelling on them.

In a randomized control trial at Rush University Medical Center in Chicago, adults with chronic insomnia who tried the practice for eight weeks slept better.[13]

Try it yourself, like this:

- If a thought or worry is whirling around your mind at bedtime, acknowledge that it's there but don't dwell on it or add to it any judgments such as "I'm so silly to think that" or "I'm annoyed with myself for feeling so upset." Instead, bring your attention back to the here and now by concentrating on your breathing. You might want to use a phrase to help you focus—something like "Breathe in the calm, breathe out the stress" can help.
- Breathe in slowly, imagining the calm flooding your body and mind; then on your exhale, imagine seeing the air you breathe out travel away from you, carrying with it your internal stress.

✦ As you breathe this way, while thoughts are forcing their way into your mind, simply keep acknowledging them and tell your-self you'll deal with them at another, more appropriate, time. Then bring your attention back to your breathing.

You can learn how to do mindfulness meditation via apps, or take a mindfulness class online or in your area.

56 ✦ See thoughts as passing clouds

It can also be helpful to imagine any anxious thoughts that come into your head as passing clouds, drifting across the sky. This helps you see those thoughts as any observer would see them, separate from you. Imagine you're lying in a warm field, on a picnic blanket in the grass. You're comfortable and sleepy and there's a warm breeze gently fanning you, a scent of flowers, and the distant hum of bees. It's a beautiful sunny day, with a few clouds in a blue sky.

As a thought enters your mind, give it a name—worry, sadness, anxiety, fear—and place it in a fluffy white cloud. As it passes across the sky you can choose to linger on it, or you can simply observe the thought, acknowledge it, and let it drift by and dissipate.

This practice helps you realize you can choose how to react to unhelpful thoughts: engage with them or let them pass.

57 ✦ Keep a calming note card by your bed

Therapists often advise people prone to anxiety or panic attacks to keep coping or calming note cards on them to pull out whenever they feel overwhelmed. Similarly, if you often wake at night feeling panic, or experience anxiety when you're lying in bed trying to drop off, it can be handy to write out and keep a calming card on your bedside table. Use an index card or similar. Write on it reassuring, true information with the aim of replacing the anxious feelings you may be having with more relaxed and balanced thoughts.

If you're prone to panic attacks, statements you may want to write on the cards could include "This is uncomfortable but I am safe and the feelings will pass," "I have been through this before and I have survived," "I can get through this." If you're prone to anxious thoughts, try using statements like "These are just thoughts, not realities," and "Worrying doesn't help."

Keep the statements short so you can perhaps repeat them like a mantra when you reach for the card in the night. If possible, read them out loud (again, if there's someone in bed with you this may not be practical!) and remember to breathe deeply and slowly.

58 ✦ Get an earful of Nature

Listening to familiar natural sounds, such as the wind in the trees or rainfall, can help alter connections in our brains and switch our minds and bodies from fight-or-flight mode to rest-and-digest mode, a sign of relaxation.

Researchers from Brighton and Sussex Medical School in the UK rounded up a group of volunteers and played them sounds recorded from either natural or artificial environments while measuring their brain and nervous-system activity. They found that when the volunteers listened to the natural sounds in a state of stress, their bodies relaxed and their brains veered away from inward-focused thinking, which is associated with stress, anxiety and depression.[14]

There are plenty of apps and downloads of nature sounds that could help your mind wander off and send you to sleep. You can choose to be serenaded by everything from frogs at nighttime to a rolling thunderstorm or calming tropical rain. Just search the Internet for "sounds from nature relaxing apps" or similar.

59 ✦ Touch your forehead to feel less stressed

You've probably used kinesiology's emotional-stress-release technique without realizing it, when you've been worried, anxious or trying to solve a problem. It involves touching two points on your forehead, about halfway between your eyebrows and your hairline, where you may feel obvious bumps. It's the classic "I'm thinking" pose. But it also has a calming effect.

Try it. Using the tips of your fingers to touch these points, let the palms of your hands rest lightly on your closed eyes and your cheeks. The touch is thought to help attract blood to the frontal lobe area of your brain, responsible for reasoning and problem solving. It's also a part of the brain that's activated during meditation.

As you touch the points on your forehead, think about the issue that's causing you stress. Think of it in as much detail as you can, engaging all your senses if possible. What can you hear, see, taste, feel, and smell? Breathe deeply. After a while you may find your mind wandering and feel less agitated about the problem—and you may even have come up with a solution. Even if the problem is still there, though, you may perceive it differently and so it will cause you less stress.

60 ✦ Cool your brow

To get to sleep, our brains need to settle down and be calm.

Brain-imaging scans have shown that insomniacs often have a lot going on in the frontal cortex region of the brain—responsible for a racing mind, worry, and mental chatter, which makes it difficult to drop off and enjoy deep sleep. Remarkably, researchers at the University of Pittsburgh found that cooling this part of the brain can reduce metabolic activity there.[15] They gave insomniacs a cooling cap to wear that made them fall asleep sooner than those in the study who had no sleep problems. They also slept for 89 percent of the time they were in bed—the same amount as the normal sleepers.

If you find it hard to shut off your mind, try using a cold flannel compress on your forehead to see if you can put your thoughts on ice—and sleep better as a result.

61 ✦ Time to sack your sleep tracker?

Tracking your sleep using a wearable device has become de rigueur for some, but a study published in 2017 has warned it could actually make your slumber suffer.[16] The researchers discovered a new sleep disorder linked to sleep tracking that they've named "orthosomnia"—an obsession with getting correct sleep. And it's causing even normally good sleepers to be so preoccupied with tracking their z's and achieving the perfect eight hours that it causes them anxiety and—you've guessed it—sleepless nights.

A few things to bear in mind. If you're already anxious about not getting to sleep and you feel that your tracker is exacerbating the angst, get rid of it. Plus, if you wake in the night and are obsessively checking the tracker, then worrying about the readings and subsequently lying awake, stressing . . . again, throw it away! Also worth noting is that the claims of some of these devices often outweigh the science to support them—so the readings aren't always a completely accurate representation of how you've slept. If your tracker says you slept badly but you feel refreshed and energized, listen to your body rather than to the stats.

On a more positive note, trackers can be handy for those insomniacs who think they sleep far less than they do. And apparently there are lots of us. A study review published in the journal *Behaviour Research and Therapy* suggests that around a third of those who complained of insomnia didn't have particularly poor sleep when it was measured by actigraph (a device used to monitor sleep and track wakefulness).[17] Having insomnia identity, though, makes these people wake up fatigued, anxious, and depressed—as though they really do suffer terrible sleep. Another study found that showing insomniacs data from an actigraph, revealing that they had slept better than they thought, meant they felt less anxious and preoccupied with sleep the following night.[18]

Less anxiety means better sleep—so your tracker could be a sleep booster rather than a sleep stealer if it helps you in this way. You decide.

62 ✦ Accept your sleeplessness

Have you ever been ensnared by one of those tricky Chinese finger traps? The more you try to pull your fingers apart and wrestle your way out of it, the tighter the bamboo webbing constricts around your fingers. But what happens if you do the opposite to what your instincts tell you? That is, give up the fight with the trap by gently relaxing your fingers, bringing them together rather than trying to prise them apart—and it's easier to break free.

It's the same with insomnia. Battle against it, and you'll experience not only the unpleasantness of being awake but yet nastier sensations like anger, frustration, or panic, which will make sleep extra elusive. Accept it, make peace with it, and stop struggling, however, and—paradoxically—you're more likely to win the contest and consequently get better sleep. More and more sleep therapists are encouraging "insomnia acceptance" among patients as a way of overcoming their sleep problems. This involves relaxing into your sleeplessness, not railing against it, and replacing your negative reactions (the panic, worry, anger, and frustration) with positive ones.

Try remembering the following pointers if you can't get to sleep:

- Yes, you may be awake now, but everyone, including you, is capable of sleep, and it will come.
- Be confident that everyone gets sleepy at some point—and that you will, too.
- Don't fear not sleeping—tell yourself that everyone sleeps; it might take you a long time but you will sleep eventually.
- Remind yourself that the fact you are resting in bed, even if you're not sleeping, will do your body good and help you cope well the following day.
- Reassure yourself that a few hours of sleeplessness will do you no great harm.

Accept your sleeplessness, and you'll come to realize that much of the unpleasantness you associate with not sleeping is generated by your frustration and anger as you rail against it. In other words, it's not being awake that's the biggest problem: it's your emotional responses to being awake that exacerbate your insomnia.

As your negative emotions about not sleeping subside, your stress response should switch off and you may well find yourself nodding off, too.

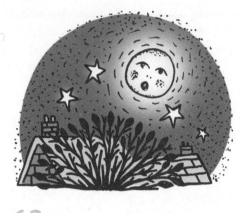

63 ✦ Be guided by imagery

Guided imagery is a relaxation technique designed to create a calm environment in your mind. It does this by helping you summon up mental images that evoke a sense of tranquility, well-being, and relaxation along with instilling perceptions of comfort, perfect warmth, and being in a safe and peaceful place.

In one hospital study 80 percent of patients who listened to an audio recording of guided imagery focusing on pain reduction, easing anxiety, and promoting sleep said that it helped in some way.[19] You can download recordings or apps of guided imagery that can help transport you to anything from a powder-white tropical beach to a peaceful English meadow, to watching stars appear in the night sky or even swimming with dolphins. Or you might want to imagine yourself lying in a canoe on a calm lake, looking up at a clear blue sky; or snuggled in a black velvet hammock in a completely dark room. Both are techniques that were reportedly used by the US military in World War II to help aviators fall asleep fast!

64 ✦ Cultivate a beginner's mind— see every night as new

"Beginner's mind," or *shoshin,* is a way of thinking that comes from Zen Buddhism. It encourages you to look at things as if seeing and experiencing them for the first time, free from any preconceptions or baggage. It's a way of thinking that's not burdened by experience and one that's ready to learn afresh. It's the opposite of "expert mind," which we adopt when we've done something often enough to believe that we don't need to question how we do it. We do it automatically, believing that it's the right—or only—way to do it.

Some psychologists say that many insomniacs have adopted an expert mind as regards their way of trying to sleep. They have come to believe that their body simply doesn't know how to sleep well and that it's something they are cursed with. They may believe the only thing that can help them is sleeping pills or other crutches such as alcohol, and that there's no point in trying something new. Mindfulness-based therapy for insomnia often uses the concept of beginner's mind to attempt to challenge poor sleepers' assumptions about sleep and to get them to see they can start all over again and sleep well.

It works like this:

First, go to bed every night with a beginner's mind—in other words, an open mind. See each night as completely new and unique, and disregard any thoughts about how it's going to pan out compared to other nights. Try telling yourself, "This is a new night. It doesn't matter what happened last night and there's no point in worrying about what I need to do tomorrow. I will approach this night with a fresh mind as to what will happen, not with dread."

Try to abandon your preconceived ideas about sleep—"My body can't sleep well," "I'm going to feel terrible tomorrow," "The health consequences for me will be awful"—and to start afresh with a new approach: one that includes the fact that everyone can (and does) sleep and that your body has the ability to do it if you let it. Try telling yourself, "My body and mind can sleep well if I let them. I trust that they can do this naturally. It's not helpful to worry and feel anxious. My body and mind want to help me. It doesn't matter if I don't get seven or eight hours. Rest is important to me so I will enjoy this relaxation. I will trust my own ability to let go and get to sleep." Then it's a case of opening your mind to the here and now: no past worries about not being able to sleep, and no future worries about being tired tomorrow. Lie in bed comfortably, mindful of the sensations you feel: your heartbeat and breathing, the air filling your nose, how each part of your body feels from head to toe.

You can cultivate a beginner's mind in other ways, with some simple mindfulness exercises such as taking an everyday object and looking at it as if you've never seen it before. Many mindfulness teachers suggest choosing a raisin as an example—look, touch, smell, and taste it as if it's completely new to you.

Try walking around your town and looking up from time to time—you'll probably see some amazing architecture you've never noticed before. Or take up a new hobby or learn a new skill. Testing out new ways of using your beginner's mind could lead you to look at your sleep in a new way.

65 ✦ Give your mind a pleasurable task

Various sleep studies have found that "cognitive distraction"—diverting your mind from worrying to pleasant thoughts—can help you get better sleep.[20] One interesting way to do this is to give your mind an enjoyable but not too taxing task to do as you lie in bed. Maybe imagine how you'd decorate a room in your house, how you'd landscape your garden if you have one, or how you'd make the shed into a game room. Imagine the colors and tones of the paint you'd use, the feel and texture of the fabrics, the colors and scents of flowers and foliage.

The scene needs to be compelling enough to take your mind off worry, but not so exciting that it keeps you awake.

66 ✦ Talk about yourself

If worries are stopping you from nodding off, then talking about yourself, out loud or in your head, may be effective. But it has to be in the third person.

Researchers at Michigan State University and the University of Michigan carried out studies showing individuals upsetting photographs and asking others to recall painful experiences.[21]

The participants' brain activity was measured after this unpleasant exposure, and, in both cases, when they referred to themselves in the third person using their names rather than the first person "I," emotional brain activity quickly decreased. The researchers surmised that talking about yourself as "he" or "she" helps you think about yourself more like you think about others, permitting you to gain a little psychological distance from what's worrying or distressing you. And that can help you regulate your emotions and see things more clearly and calmly.

So, for example, I might say to myself, "Kim is really worried she's going to botch the presentation at work tomorrow." Or "Kim is feeling really fed up because she knows she won't get to sleep for hours." When I talk like this I'm more likely to be able to analyze my emotions better, and with less bias. I can see my worries from a different perspective—in a more measured way. All of which could contribute to calming me and making me see that I may be over-reacting, overruminating and overworrying.

67 ✦ Hypnotize yourself to sleep

Look into my eyes. Now watch my swinging pocket watch. You are feeling sleepy . . .

Forget the mysterious, old-fashioned quackery impression of hypnotism you may have gleaned from watching too many old Hollywood films. It's moved on since the dark old days. Now there are hypnotherapy apps and YouTube videos to watch that could help you set the stage for a great night's slumber.

Sleep hypnosis encourages you to concentrate on someone speaking specific soothing verbal cues, and it can draw you away from any anxieties that may stop you from sleeping, relax your mind and body, and ease you into a trance-like state, or even into a deeper, slow-wave sleep (SWS)—the sort that's really restorative—helping repair your immune system and consolidate memories.

In a study published in the scientific journal *Sleep*, researchers from two German universities asked women to listen to two thirteen-minute recordings on two occasions before going to sleep.[22] One was a tape containing hypnotic suggestions to "sleep deeper," using the metaphor of a fish swimming deeper and deeper into water. The other—control—tape was a documentary on mineral deposits.

Brain-wave activity was measured, and it was found that when the women listened to the hypnosis tape they enjoyed 81 percent more deep, slow-wave sleep and spent 67 percent less time awake than when they'd listened to the other, neutral, tape.

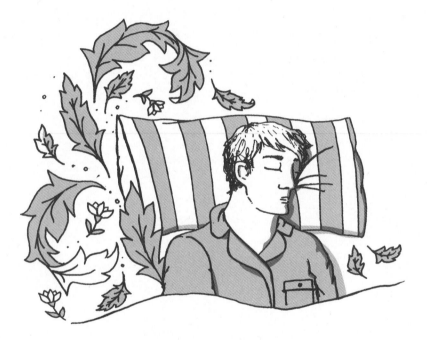

Three

Bedroom Tricks

Your bedroom needs to be a breathing space and a haven from the outside world—a place you associate with rest, calm, and comfort, and one you look forward to heading off to at the end of the day for some much-needed nestling down. The tips and tricks in this chapter will help you create a space that cocoons you in an ambience of serene tranquility—one that will woo you to dreamland. Night night.

68 ✦ Keep yourself in the dark

Your bedroom has to be pretty dark for you to fall asleep easily—and stay asleep. As I explained earlier, darkness triggers the release of melatonin, the hormone that promotes restful sleep; and even a small amount of light hitting the cells in our retinas—from a street light, for example—can hamper its production.

When you turn out the light, you shouldn't be able to see your hand clearly in front of your face. After your eyes have gotten used to the dark, you should still find it difficult to see across the room.

69 ✦ Work out how the light gets in

If your room isn't pitch black, look for where the light is leaking in and fix that leak. If it's seeping in through your curtains, try lined or blackout curtains, or blinds. A good old-fashioned draft stopper can prevent any light from creeping in at the bottom of the door. And close the door if light from the rest of the house, from the landing or hall perhaps, is coming into your bedroom.

70 ✦ Turn it off

Who knew that even the small amount of light emitted by your phone, a charging iPad, or your radio can disturb your sleep? Switch off all your appliances or cover them up when you turn out the bedroom light. Opt for digital radios or clocks that have orange or red light displays rather than those with sleep-disrupting white or blue light, if you can.

71 ✦ Cover clock faces . . .

. . . or turn timepieces away from you when you switch off the lights. Why? Because if you start clock-watching when you can't sleep you'll start stressing out about how much sleep you're missing. Then you'll start counting how many hours you have left until your alarm goes off. Then you'll start to worry about how badly you'll cope tomorrow. In short, by now your mind will be busy and anxious, which will keep you awake for even longer.

So as soon as you've set your alarm, turn it away from eye's view.

72 ✦ Get your night-light right, and go red

If you use night-lights in your bedroom—maybe they make you feel safer, or you use them to line your route to the bathroom for nighttime trips so you don't trip up—you might want to change them for the red-bulbed variety. Even the dim light from a white or blue night-light can interrupt melatonin secretion. Red-based light has a longer wavelength and less power to interfere with your sleepy state. So go red.

73 ✦ Don't use your phone as your alarm clock

If your phone is the last thing you look at before lights-out and the first thing you look at in the morning, it can lead to unhealthy habits. When you set your phone's alarm at night, for instance, does it often turn into a quick check of those emails or social media? An hour later, are you wound up by work worries or hyped up by a Twitter storm? Plus, there's the issue of all that blue light confusing your body's circadian clock, so you may end up feeling wide awake again.

Get a proper alarm clock, or use one on a radio, making sure the alarm tone is a gentle one—not a loud ring, which can jolt you out of sleep with a shock. Leave your phone out of the bedroom, or at least out of arm's reach. And checking emails or social media is not the most relaxing way to start your day—is it what you end up doing when you switch off your phone's morning alarm? Be honest.

74 ✦ Play around with your pillows!

Are you a side sleeper, or do you prefer to sleep flat on your back? Or perhaps you like to lie on your front? Any position has the potential to put strain on your back, which can stop you from falling asleep or make you wake up intermittently through the night. The good news? Pillows aren't just for heads—you can position them strategically elsewhere to help prevent back pain.

If you're a stomach sleeper, try popping a pillow under your lower abdomen and pelvis to take some pressure off your back. Use a flattish pillow, or none, for your head. If you sleep on your side, try drawing your legs slightly toward your chest and placing a pillow between your knees to keep your hips, pelvis, and spine aligned. If you like to sleep on your back, put a pillow under your knees.

There. Perfect pillow placement for all!

75 ✦ Ache when you wake?

If you toss and turn to get comfy at lights-out, wake up in the early hours feeling sore, or ache when you wake, your mattress may be to blame.

But is it too hard or too soft? If your mattress is too hard, physiotherapists generally say you'll be more likely to feel pain at pressure points such as the hips, pelvis, or shoulder. If it's too soft and unsupportive, you might feel discomfort in the neck, shoulder, or mid or lower back.

So be like Goldilocks and find a mattress that's not too hard, not too soft—but just right for you.

76 ✦ Mattress lost its mojo?

Whatever the case, mattresses do start to degrade after seven to ten years—or even earlier if they're not of good quality. So it may be time for a new one if you want a comfortable night's sleep.

One Oklahoma State University study took a group of healthy volunteers who were sleeping on mattresses that were on average nine and a half years old and who were experiencing back pain and disturbed sleep. The study leaders outfitted them with new medium-firm mattresses for twenty-eight days, and guess what? The volunteers reported better sleep and less painful backs.[1]

77 ✦ Lie back and relax . . . at the mattress store

Buying a new mattress is one of the most important purchases you're going to make. So it makes sense that you don't rush into it, or feel pressured, when you're shopping for one. Don't be shy about lying on as many beds as you like in the store—in your preferred sleeping position, front, back, or side—for several minutes at a time to get a real feel of how comfortable they are.

Remember these tricks:

- If you're a back sleeper, the mattress should support you enough that the natural "S" curve of your spine remains when you lie down. Slide your hand flat, palm downward, under the small of your back. If you struggle to get your hand there, the mattress is probably too soft because your back is "rounding," and if there's a big gap for your hand to move around, then it's too firm and not supporting your back. Ideally your hand should slide under your back and fit snugly there, still touching it.

- If you lie on your side, your spine should stay straight—as it would be when you stand up straight. Get your partner or a friend to check.

78 ✦ Pillow-perfect

Our heads are pretty heavy. They weigh between ten and fourteen pounds, and place quite a burden on our neck muscles. It's important, therefore, to find pillows that properly support our heads while we sleep so that we don't wake with a real pain in the neck! A supportive pillow should keep your head and neck in line with your spine, just as they would be when you are standing. To check that your pillow is accurately doing its job, try these tricks:

- If you're a side sleeper, bring the hand closest to the bed under your neck, feeling for any upward or downward tilt. An upward tilt and the pillow is too high, a downward tilt and it's too low for you. The pillow should be just the right size to fill the gap between the top of your shoulder and your head.
- If you're a back sleeper, place your hand on the back of your neck to feel for any forward or backward tilt. Your forehead and chin should be level.
- Sleeping on your front is the worst position for neck pain, and most experts agree if you really have to sleep like this then try sleeping without a pillow.

If you persistently suffer from neck pain in bed, you might want to try an orthopedic pillow. One study found they helped support the neck and maintain the cervical curve better than feather or memory-foam pillows.[2]

You could also try visiting a physiotherapy practice that offers a service where they can measure you for a perfect-fit pillow.

79 ✦ Is your bed big enough?

Size matters when it comes to getting a good night's sleep, especially if you share your bed with a partner. The average person will move around up to sixty or seventy times a night, so you're bound to be disturbed by a restless sleeper in a small bed. Bear in mind that a standard double bed is about four-feet, six-inches wide, giving each partner less space than a single bed, which is about three feet wide. It's best to go for a bed as big as you can afford and that your room size allows. The Sleep Council suggests doing this test with your bed partner: lie side by side, with your arms behind your head and your elbows out. If your elbows touch, your bed isn't wide enough.

Your bed should also be about four to six inches longer than the tallest person sleeping in it. A standard double bed measures about six-feet, three-inches long and a king size is about six-feet, six-inches. If you're tall you should choose a bed frame without a raised foot-board so you don't end up feeling cramped—and with stubbed toes! If you're really tall then look for companies that make extra-long beds … they are out there, but can cost a lot. And get this for a fun fact: you actually grow in height overnight as your spinal discs decompress when you lie down! So allow for an extra inch or two!

80 ✦ A game of two halves

Are you always on the losing side in the duvet tug-of-war and end up out in the cold? Or perhaps it's you who rolls yourself up snug as a bug as your other half huffs and puffs trying to pull their half of the duvet back?

Whatever the case, the solution could be to sleep like the Scandinavians do. With *two* duvets. One single duvet each. It makes complete sense in that not only do you get to keep covered and cozy—and less likely to wake in the night because you're cold—but you can also choose a warmer or cooler duvet than your sleeping partner prefers.

Simple solution! But it could be key to an undisturbed night's sleep. And if you're worried two duvets on the bed will look messy the morning after, just drape a blanket or throw over them both. Neat.

Alternatively, you could buy a duvet that's larger than strictly necessary. If you sleep in a standard double bed, buy a king-size duvet. If you sleep in a king-size bed, buy a California king–size one. That way neither of you ends up uncovered in the middle-of-the-night duvet fight.

81 ✦ Let sleeping dogs lie?

We've all been told that letting man's best friend sleep in the bedroom can disturb your own sleep. But research from the Mayo Clinic might have some good news for your cuddle-mutt.[3]

In the study, adults and their dogs wore activity trackers to monitor sleeping habits when the dog slept in the bedroom. Results showed that letting a furry family member on the bed and under the covers did, indeed, disrupt the adults' sleep quality. But the good news for devoted dog owners is this: you don't actually need to ban your canine companion from the bedroom completely. The same study found that allowing a dog to sleep *off* the bed—say, on the floor at the foot of it—didn't necessarily adversely affect its owner's sleep.

So, if you find it a comfort—or feel safer—with your dog in the bedroom, then it's fine to let a sleeping dog lie (on the floor). However, if your dog is restless and you're aware that it wakes you during the night, then you have to be firm with Fido and put him to bed downstairs.

82 ✦ Drop a few degrees

The body's core temperature needs to fall by about 2 degrees Fahrenheit in order for our brains to receive the message to initiate the surge in nighttime melatonin production that helps us fall asleep. Years ago—before so many of our homes were centrally heated and insulated—our bodies would more naturally experience this gradual dip in core body temperature that comes as the sun sets. But now that we're cocooned in unnaturally warm environments, it can be hard to cool off. Our brains, therefore, might not easily receive those essential messages to pump out the sleep hormones.

The ideal bedroom temperature is about 65 degrees Fahrenheit. Check yours—you'll probably find it's higher than that, so think about dropping your thermostat, turning off radiators in your bedroom, or letting in a little outside air.

83 ✦ Cool it on hot days

During bouts of hot weather, even the best of sleepers can struggle to fall asleep and stay asleep.

On hot sunny days keep your bedroom as cool as you can by drawing the curtains and shutting blinds throughout the day to keep the sun out. Open the windows at the front and back of the house to allow any air to circulate, and open windows at the top of the house—warm air rises, so this will give it an escape route.

Use an electric fan to circulate the air and place a bowl of ice cubes in front of it to cool the air as it blows.

84 ✦ Pave a way

Every night, check that the route from your bed to the bathroom is totally clear of any obstacles you could trip over if you need to visit the bathroom at night. That's because, when you do wake up, you should avoid switching on any lights, which can mess with your melatonin production—and make you feel more awake.

Keep in the dark to stay as sleepy as you can, with your eyes half-open, half-closed—without putting yourself in any danger, of course! Keep a dim flashlight by the bed if you really can't see where you're going.

85 ✦ A clean sheet

Are you washing your bed sheets weekly?

Well, you should be. Bed linen not only soaks up sweat and body oils but also harbors dead skin cells: perfect food for dust mites, which can cause allergies—and disturb sleep.

A poll by the National Sleep Foundation found that 71 percent of people had a more comfortable night's sleep on clean sheets, and 29 percent even headed off to bed earlier when they'd put fresh-smelling sheets on their beds.[4] So wash yours weekly at a high temperature. No excuses.

86 ✦ Listen to white—or pink—noise

If traffic, neighbors, dogs barking, your other half snoring, or other bothersome noises stop you from falling, and staying, asleep you might want to try listening to white or pink noise. This kind of unchanging, constant background noise (such as rainfall, or the sound of a vacuum cleaner or a fan) contains lots of frequencies of equal intensity and helps mask or block out the environmental noise around you.

A study published in *Frontiers in Human Neuroscience* found that people who were played pink noise—a mix of high and low frequencies that sounds a little like a waterfall—enjoyed more slow-wave or deep sleep.[5] And in an article published in the journal *Sleep* researchers noted that participants in their study fell asleep about 40 percent faster when listening to white noise.[6]

You can buy white- and pink-noise apps featuring things like ocean waves, or even the washing machine, to listen to at bedtime.

Alternatively, simply switch on a radio. Tuning in to a talk show or similar can help distract you from noise outside and relax your mind. As long as you don't find the content too riveting, it could help you nod off.

87 ✦ Plump for natural fibers

Your sheets could be interfering with the quality of your sleep. Synthetic materials such as polyester don't absorb moisture well and, as most of us perspire a little during the night—some more than others, especially if you're going through menopause—this means we're lying in our own sweat, which can be pretty uncomfortable.

So go for natural materials like cotton, which are breathable. They not only absorb the moisture from your skin but also release it by evaporation, keeping you drier and more comfortable. The same goes for your duvet and pillows. Choose a natural filling such as wool, silk, or down rather than synthetic.

88 ✦ Keep a blanket, slippers, and robe by the bed

We've established that your bedroom needs to be quite cool to help you fall asleep (around 65 degrees Fahrenheit). But, because our body temperature falls during the night, reaching its lowest at about 3:00 or 4:00 AM, if your bedroom is too chilly and your bed linen too light, you may wake up around that time because you're shivering.

For this reason, keep an extra blanket by the side of the bed that you can drowsily drape over you if you do wake up. This may be enough to coax you back to sleep. Similarly, if you wake needing the bathroom, have your slippers and robe within easy reach, to keep you warm on your trip to the bathroom.

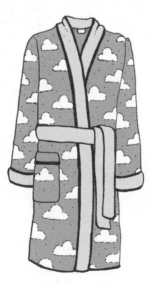

89 ✦ Use a weighted blanket

A Swedish study published in the *Journal of Sleep Medicine and Disorders* found that insomniacs who were given weighted blankets to sleep under found it easier to settle down to sleep, enjoyed calmer, better slumber through the night, and woke feeling more refreshed.[7]

Weighted blankets are usually filled with plastic pellets to make them heavy. You can buy these blankets online and it's recommended you go for one that's about 10 percent of your body weight. It's thought that the deep touch pressure, or evenly distributed weight, mimics the feeling of being hugged or massaged, helping raise your output of serotonin (which contributes to the production of melatonin) and calm the nervous system.

Best to check with your doctor before buying a weighted blanket in case it might interfere with your circulation or breathing. Or experiment with using an extra blanket over your duvet, for a similar effect.

90 ✦ Make your bed . . . but not first thing

A poll by the National Sleep Foundation found that people who make their beds every day are 19 percent more likely to get a good night's sleep than those who don't bother. It makes sense. A messy heap of tangled sheets and a lumpy duvet are uncomfortable. A neat, tidy bed invites you to sink into it. You choose.

So yes, make your bed. But here's some good advice from scientists at Kingston University: don't do it as soon as you get up.[8]

Instead, pull back the sheets and let your bed breathe. Allergy- and asthma-causing house dust mites thrive in our beds, feeding off the skin cells we shed and absorbing moisture from our sweat. If you make your bed as soon as you wake, you're keeping the covers and the mattress nice and moist for the little critters.

So leave it unmade and let light and air get to the sheets to remove the moisture, so that the mites dehydrate and eventually die. After letting the bed breathe for a while, just make sure you make it and neaten it up before bedtime.

91 ✦ Create a biophilic bedroom

Biophilic design, which uses aspects of nature and the natural world, is a big trend in both architecture and interior design. It comes as more health experts realize how much our physical and mental well-being can benefit from our connections with nature, and that being cooped up all day in built-up artificial spaces such as offices and shopping centers can drain our energies and even contribute to poor health.

It's easy to bring biophilic design into your bedroom to give both your well-being and your sleep a boost. Start with the basics and steer clear of furniture made from manmade materials if you can: go for wood instead. A study published in the *International Journal of Environmental Research and Public Health* in 2017 revealed that touching wood can slow our heart rate and reduce sympathetic-nervous activity—signs of relaxation.[9]

Hang pictures of nature on your walls. Other research has found that just looking at photos of green spaces such as woodland, grass, parks, and fields helps switch off the body's stress response.[10]

And add some houseplants to the room to clear the air for better sleep. NASA's "Clean Air Study," conducted to find the best ways to clean the air in space stations, discovered that plants such as peace lilies and chrysanthemums are pretty clever when it comes to removing common household toxins such as benzene and formaldehyde (found in synthetic fabrics and paint) from the air.[11]

92 ✦ Be more *lagom*-like

Does your bedroom exude a feeling of calm, or does it scream "Chaos!" at you? Clearing out the mess and disorder of a shambolic sleeping space and applying the Swedish principles of lagom to your bedroom could be the key to getting better shut-eye.

Swedish living spaces emit serenity and order rather than chaos and confusion thanks to the lagom way of living, which roughly translates as "just right"—not too much and not too little. Though they are homely and welcoming, they're never overloaded with unnecessary possessions or decoration. Because of this, Swedish bedrooms feel spacious, airy, fresh, and zen-like, inviting you to lie back and relax and melt away the tensions of your day.

Thus, you can achieve a more lagom-like bedroom by keeping the decor simple. Choose a neutral palette that echoes organic materials— try cool greys, beiges, and whites to create a feeling of natural airiness, then warm things up with soft cozy blankets, cushions, and bedding in similar hues. And keep decoration to a minimum. Apply the principles of lagom when you're next out shopping—think: Do you really need to buy that item? Will it take up unnecessary space?

93 ✦ Declutter!

A cluttered bedroom can put you on edge as soon as you walk into it. Not only is that pile of papers or laundry a reminder of unfinished jobs that need doing, but being bombarded by untidiness can adversely stimulate your brain, raise your cortisol level, and even feel suffocating—as if the room is closing in on you.

A psychology study from St. Lawrence University found that people who live in cluttered environments took longer to fall asleep and experienced a worse quality of sleep than people who weren't surrounded by stuff.[12] So if you want to keep clutter in check, set aside an hour to do the following:

- Ensure every surface in your bedroom has no more than three or four items on it. Your bedside table could have a lamp, a book, and a glass of water, for example, but no knick-knacks. Be strict.
- Gather everything in your room that belongs elsewhere and put it away.
- Purge and play the five-second decluttering game. Pick an item, then decide within five seconds if it's useful to you and brings

you happiness, or if it's just taking up space. Have three bags ready—one for items you'll give to charity or a friend, another for things you will sell, and the third for trash. Be ruthless and remind yourself how calming and comforting your bedroom will look with less paraphernalia in it.

✦ In short, fill your room with just the things you need and enjoy—nothing more.

94 ✦ Keep your bed a sleep-and-sex-only zone

You've probably heard this one before—but here it is again, just in case. Keep your bed just for sleep and sex. You need to build a strong association with it as a place for rest, sleep, kisses, and cuddles only. But if you're also using your bed to catch up on emails on your tablet, write work reports on your laptop, or watch an addictive show on television—all pretty stimulating things—that association with rest and pleasure is going to be pretty weak.

Remember: Your bed needs to be a refuge from rousing, thought-provoking, anxiety-inducing activities. A place to switch off.

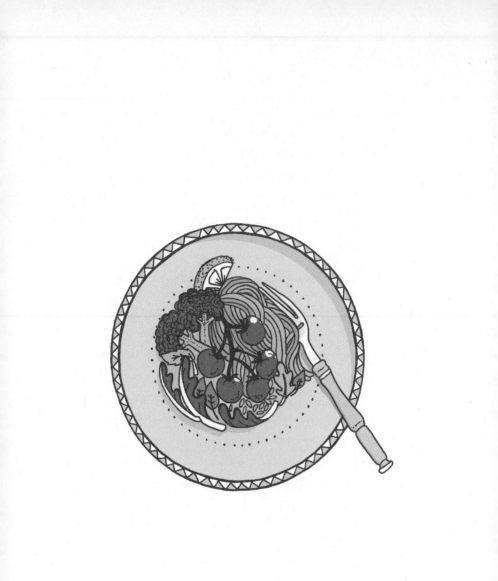

Four

Food and Drink Tips

A healthy diet impacts on everything from our weight and mood to our energy quotient and our risk of heart disease, type 2 diabetes, and even cancer. But what's less well known is that what we eat and drink can also sabotage—or support—our slumber. Fueling our bodies with the right food and drink will provide our brains with the nutrients they need to produce neurotransmitters that help maintain healthy sleep cycles.

Some foods can keep us awake, too, while others may have sleep-inducing properties. Plus, when and how much you eat can also affect how easy, or not, it may be to nod off.

Follow these food and drink tricks to ensure that what you feed yourself helps you get your forty winks—and then some.

95 ✦ Impose a caffeine curfew

Caffeine peps you up by blocking the effects of adenosine, a brain chemical thought to be involved in promoting sleep. The effects can take eight hours to fully wear off, so a cup of coffee in the late afternoon could interfere with falling asleep that night. Set yourself a coffee caffeine curfew of about 2:00 PM to ensure it's all out of your system by the time you hit the sack.

Don't forget the other caffeine culprits: tea, colas, energy drinks, and some cold and flu remedies also contain it. Even chocolate contains a small amount of the stuff (the darker the chocolate, the more caffeine). Alas, chocolate's probably not the best midnight snack . . .

96 ✦ Steer clear of too much spice

A spicy meal before bed can give you indigestion, another cause of difficulty sleeping. Research has also shown that capsaicin, the active chemical that gives chile peppers their spicy heat, can trigger the process by which cells convert energy into heat (thermogenesis) and so increase your body temperature—yet another thing that can interfere with your ability to drop off.

A study from the University of Tasmania clearly showed this effect.[1] Volunteers were served Tabasco sauce and mustard with their evening meal. Their body temperature rose, and they took longer to fall asleep than usual, had less slow-wave, deep sleep, and spent more time awake than normal.

So if you're intending to indulge in a spicy meal, you might want to eat it at lunchtime—or at least a few hours before bed so everything can cool off.

97 ✦ Go easy on greasy foods

We all know that eating too many high-fat foods can increase our risk of heart disease, obesity, and certain cancers. But fatty foods can also disrupt your sleep. A study published in 2016 in the *Journal of Clinical Sleep Medicine* found that consuming a lot of saturated fats during the day was associated with lighter, less restorative sleep and more waking up during the night.[2]

Try limiting "bad" fats like those in processed meats, pastries, cakes, and cookies and instead choose foods containing "good" heart-healthy unsaturated fats—like nuts, seeds, avocados, and oils such as olive and sunflower.

Other ways to cut back on saturated fat? Remove all the visible fat from meat and the skin from poultry, swap to reduced-fat or skim milk; and boil, steam or grill foods rather than roasting or frying them in butter, lard or coconut oil.

98 ✦ Shun too much sugar

A high-sugar diet can deprive you of sweet dreams, according to research, because the spikes and crashes in your blood sugar that you get after eating sweet foods can cause restlessness and disturb your sleep.[3]

One sugary culprit you should definitely cut back on? Sugar-sweetened caffeinated sodas. A study published in *Sleep Health* found that adults who slept for less than five hours a night consumed 21 percent more sugar-sweetened drinks than those who got seven to eight hours.[4] Interestingly, it was suggested that not only could such drinks account for impaired sleep, but also being short on sleep could make you crave more of the same.

Whatever the case, refined sugar is not good for your body, so as well as cutting back on it in all its obvious forms—candy, chocolates, desserts—look at replacing simple carbohydrates like white bread, pasta, and rice with their whole-grain equivalents.

99 ✦ Eat early

Eating too late at night will make it difficult not only to fall asleep, but to stay asleep, too. As we know, our core body temperature must fall for us to drop off. But eating makes it rise, as blood is directed toward our digestive system—our core. So aim to stop eating a few hours before bed.

You may want to consider adopting a time-restricted-eating (TRE) pattern, which just means you eat only during a certain time window, usually between six and twelve hours. One study found that people who followed a ten-hour TRE program—say between 8:00 AM and 6:00 PM—enjoyed better sleep.[5]

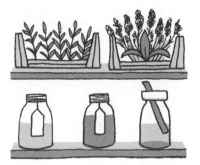

100 ✦ Eat and drink adaptogens

Adaptogens are compounds found in plants that are believed to help your body adapt to pressure and tension, possibly by regulating the release of stress hormones. They've been used in Ayurvedic medicine for centuries to help relieve anxiety. Some studies of foods and herbs from the adaptogen family, such as ginger and ashwagandha root, have confirmed their stress-busting abilities.[6]

Other foods in the family include nettles, licorice, moringa, turmeric, and maca. Look for herbal teas with these ingredients for a soothing sip before lights-out, or any time when stress threatens to take over.

101 ✦ Plenty of fruit and veggies

As the foundation of a healthy, balanced diet, eating plenty of fruits and vegetables can help reduce the risk of heart disease, stroke, and some cancers—and could help you get just the right amount of sleep, too.

A cross-sectional study using data from the National Diet and Nutrition Survey and published in the journal *BMJ Open* found that "medium sleepers," who slept for seven to eight hours a night—the amount of sleep that those who enjoy better overall health generally get—ate 24 grams more fruit and veggies than "short sleepers," who managed fewer than seven hours a night and ate 28 grams more than "long sleepers," who slept more than eight hours a night.[7] Research has shown a correlation between long sleeping and an increased mortality risk.

Figures indicate that at least two-thirds of us aren't eating the recommended five a day. To up your intake and get the optimum seven to eight hours of sleep a night, too, try starting as you mean to go on: make a habit of adding some fruit to your breakfast cereal, oatmeal, or yogurt. Then ensure you have some sort of salad in your sandwiches for lunch and have vegetable side dishes with dinner. Snack on carrot, celery, and pepper sticks through the day.

A heart-healthy Mediterranean diet has also been linked to good sleep. So eat like a Greek and fuel up with plenty of plant foods such as vegetables, whole grains, legumes, and nuts; replace butter with olive oil; and rein in the red meat.

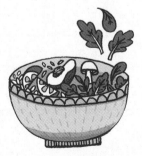

102 ✦ Don't pass on prebiotics

Prebiotics are a form of dietary fiber—found in foods like artichokes, raw garlic, leeks, and onions—that feed and contribute to the number of friendly probiotic bacteria in our gut.

But prebiotics are not only good for your tummy. Research has found that there's a chance they could improve your sleep as well as protect you from insomnia following a stressful event.[8] The study, performed on rats, found that those fed on a prebiotic diet spent more time in peaceful and restorative non-rapid-eye-movement sleep than those on a non-prebiotic diet. Also, after being exposed to a stressor, the rats on the prebiotic diet spent more time in rapid-eye-movement (REM) sleep, the type that's thought to help protect you from stress. The researchers noted that although earlier studies had suggested stress can alter gut bacteria in a way that interferes with sleep, the rats on the prebiotic diet appeared to be protected from these changes.

It's unclear exactly what role prebiotics can have on human sleep—but eating healthy sources of prebiotic fiber can't hurt.

103 ✦ Fuel up with fiber!

We should all be eating 30 grams of dietary fiber daily to help keep our digestion systems healthy. And it now seems that eating enough fiber could also help us fall asleep more easily—and get a better kind of shut-eye, too.[9] Researchers from Columbia University put a number of adults on healthy controlled diets for four days, monitoring their sleep.

For the fifth and sixth days, the recruits could eat what they wanted. In the event, the ones who ate a low-fiber diet on those last two days took longer to drift off to dreamland and had less deep sleep, too.

You can up your fiber intake by eating beans, lentils, brown rice, whole-grain breakfast cereals, whole-wheat pasta, and fruit and vegetables like apples, berries, celery, and broccoli.

104 ✦ Abstain from alcohol

That nightcap may help you to nod off, but you'll pay for it with a disturbed sleep. A review of scientific studies on the effects of alcohol found that while it acts as a sedative, helping you fall asleep faster and sleep deeply for the first half of the night, those benefits are offset by more disrupted sleep in the second half.[10]

Alcohol is broken down fairly quickly by the body and so the sedative effect wears off within hours, and you're left with a mini withdrawal or rebound effect, causing wakefulness or restlessness. You're also more likely to snore and sweat after drinking, or to have to go to the bathroom in the middle of the night. Cheers to that—not!

105 ✦ Go nuts for walnuts

You'd do well to snack on walnuts in the early evening. They contain their own source of melatonin, the University of Texas found, and eating them increases the amount of the hormone in your blood.[11]

Munch on them alone, or sprinkle on a salad or bowl of cereal.

106 ✦ Pep up your potassium levels

If you wake during the night, you may want to ponder on whether you're getting enough potassium in your diet.

The University of California, San Diego, found that potassium supplements helped individuals who normally consumed a low-potassium diet sleep more, and with fewer awakenings in the night.[12] Potassium can help reduce your blood pressure, regulate your heart-beat, and is good for muscle and bone strength, too.

You should be able to get enough from a healthy diet—good sources are baked sweet or white potatoes, bananas, white beans, avocados, and tomatoes.

107 ✦ Herbal help

The herbal remedy valerian has been used as a traditional medicine for sedation and sleep in many cultures. Various studies have indicated that people who take it have an 80 percent chance of reporting improved sleep compared with patients taking a placebo.[13] Evidence suggests it helps stop the breakdown of GABA (gamma-aminobutyric acid), a neurotransmitter that promotes relaxation, in the brain.

It's best to try all sorts of lifestyle measures before you take valerian, though, and do check with your doctor that it's safe for you and that it won't affect the action of any other medicines you're taking.

You could also try valerian tea, available widely.

108 ✦ Take in more tryptophan

It seems that eating foods containing tryptophan can also improve sleep.[14] It's an amino acid that's transformed into serotonin, then converted into melatonin in the body. Foods high in tryptophan include milk, poultry, and eggs.

But here's the catch: These foods contain other amino acids that compete with tryptophan to get absorbed across the blood–brain barrier. Evidence suggests, though, that combining a tryptophan-rich food with some carbohydrate can mitigate this, because the insulin that's released as a result of consuming the carbs helps decrease the amounts of these other amino acids in the blood.[15] With less competition, it's easier for tryptophan to cross the blood–brain barrier.

A good suppertime snack a few hours before bedtime, therefore, might be some low-sugar whole-grain cereal with milk.

109 ✦ Go cherry-picking

An article published in the *American Journal of Therapeutics* suggests that sipping cherry juice could help you sleep better.[16] In this small study, adults aged fifty-plus with chronic insomnia who drank two daily glasses of Montmorency tart cherry juice for two weeks (one in the morning and the other in the evening) slept on average eighty-four minutes longer and had better sleep than when they drank a placebo made to look and taste like cherry juice (but without its polyphenols) for another two weeks.

The combination of melatonin, the amino acid tryptophan, and the red-pigment proanthocyanidins in the cherries may well contribute to achieving a good night's sleep.

Cheers to cherries!

110 ✦ Eat two kiwis

Kiwi fruit aren't just bursting with vitamin C and fiber; they could also be a superfood for sleep. Scientists at Taiwan's Taipei Medical University gave some poor sleepers two kiwis to eat an hour before bedtime for four weeks, and the results were pretty sweet![17]

The study participants fell asleep more quickly and slept longer and more soundly. It could be the super-high folate and antioxidant content of the fruits that aid sleep. Low levels of both are associated with insomnia—and low levels of folate are also associated with restless legs syndrome (see page 33).

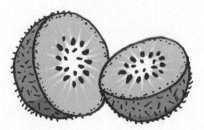

111 ✦ Go green

If you're looking for an alternative to coffee to drink during the day, go for green tea. It contains the amino acid theanine, which possesses anti-stress effects.

Make sure you go for a low-caffeine or decaffeinated green tea, though. Caffeine suppresses the anti-stress effect and, of course, too much caffeine consumed in the daytime can keep you awake at night. A couple of Japanese studies have found that drinking low-caffeine green tea during the day not only lowered stress but improved the participants' quality of sleep.[18]

112 ✦ Eat more magnesium

The mineral magnesium is important for maintaining a healthy amount of GABA (gamma-aminobutyric acid) in the body; as we mentioned earlier, GABA is a neurotransmitter that promotes relaxation.

Magnesium deficiency is associated with anxiety and stress. One study found that upping magnesium intake led to falling asleep faster, with better sleep throughout the night.[19] Magnesium is also thought to help with the symptoms of restless legs syndrome.

Good sources of magnesium are dark leafy greens, seeds and nuts, fish, and whole grains such as whole-wheat bread and brown rice. Try a brown rice pilaf with spinach, cashews, and almonds for dinner, perhaps.

113 ✦ Sip some passionflower tea

A warm drink before bed can be calming, but you may want to swap your cocoa or hot chocolate for some passionflower tea instead. An Australian university study found that people with mild sleeping difficulties who drank it for seven days slept significantly better than when they drank a placebo tea made from parsley.[20]

You can buy passionflower teabags, or dried passionflower to brew your own cup, from most health-food shops.

114 ✦ Oily fish is good for you

A study published in the *Journal of Clinical Sleep Medicine* found that eating fatty fish such as salmon can have a positive impact on your sleep.[21] Oily fish is high in vitamin D and essential omega-3 fatty acids, and is also thought to play a role in protecting against heart disease. Health guidelines suggest we should eat at least two portions of fish each week, at least one of which should be salmon, mackerel, sardines, or trout.

So don't be a fish out of water and forgo fatty fish. Try swapping your usual chicken, pork, or beef for salmon, or flake some smoked mackerel over a salad.

Because oily fish can contain pollutants, though, we should eat no more than four portions a week (or two if you're planning a pregnancy, are pregnant, or are breastfeeding).

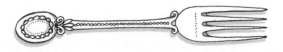

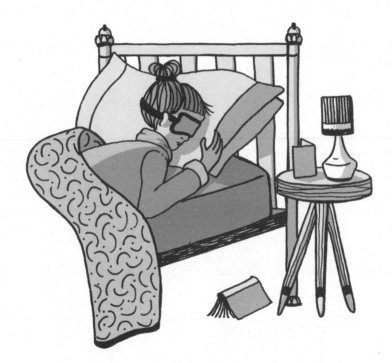

Five

Body Tricks

You know that your body needs to be tired, but relaxed, to fall asleep easily.

The trouble is that many of us get stressed during the day, and we hold that anxiety in our bodies. Our muscles tense up, leading to headaches, neck and back pain, stiffness, and even knots and spasms. So by the time you get to bed, your body may feel fidgety or like a coiled spring in gridlock—tense and tight and unable to unwind.

Follow our body tricks and techniques to help loosen your limbs, relieve the tension in your muscles, and ease your body into a state of blissful repose so you can slip more easily into slumber.

115 ✦ Force a sleepy face and fake a yawn

The "facial feedback hypothesis" in psychology says that making certain expressions can influence our emotions and how we feel generally. The theory is that mimicking a sleepy face with heavy eyelids and faking a few small yawns—just by opening your mouth wide into a yawn shape but without taking in large gulps of air, as this could actually make you feel more alert—can send your mind the message that you're tired.

Alternatively, just think about yawning—or picture people yawning around you. Studies have found that yawning is somehow contagious and that hearing, seeing, reading, or just thinking about yawning can activate mirror neurons in the brain that make us do the same thing![1]

There are plenty of videos available on the Internet that challenge you not to yawn while watching them.

116 ◆ Stick out your tongue!

Many of us hold stress in our jaw; when we feel anxious we unwittingly clench our teeth, and this can send signals of distress to our brains that make us tense up even more.

"Lion's breath" is a yoga move that can help to loosen your jaw and ease anxiety. Prepare to look crazy and wild—but don't worry, no one can see you in the dark! If you're lying in bed and notice your jaw is tense, try this trick:

◆ Inhale through your nose.
◆ On the exhale, stick out your tongue, pointing it down to your chin, and raise your eyes.
◆ Repeat five times, and you should feel your jaw loosen—and the rest of your body should follow suit.

117 ✦ Roll your eyes upward

Close your eyes, inhale, and look up to your third eye—the point between your eyebrows. Lower your eyes as you exhale and repeat four times. As you're nodding off, your eyes naturally roll upward like this to an angle of around 20 degrees. The movement is said to slow down your beta brain waves (the active ones) to the more relaxed alpha brain waves that induce sleep.

118 ✦ Give yourself a sleep signal

When you're feeling relaxed and almost drifting off, try giving your-self a physical sleep signal that will help elicit sleep when you're next having trouble nodding off. Choose something calming like putting your hand on your cheek or gently stroking your earlobe or lips.

If you repeat this exercise over successive nights when you're sleeping well, your body will learn to associate it with sleep, and next time you're having trouble nodding off, simply repeating the movement should convince your body it's sleepy.

119 ✦ Find peace with palming

This Tibetan yogic tradition is said to help calm your nervous system by relaxing your optic nerve.

First, rub your hands together to generate heat. Then place your cupped palms over your closed eyes—be careful to apply no pressure.

The heel of your hands should be resting on your cheekbones so that the palms are not touching your eyes. Breathe slowly and enjoy the feeling of the heat from your hands as it reaches your eyes.

120 ✦ Squeeze yourself to sleep

We know that our bodies have to be tension-free to fall asleep. But trying to relax all our muscles and body bits is easier said than done if we're feeling uptight.

A good technique? Squeeze, then release. Squeezing muscle groups for about five seconds at a time, then releasing them, can really help stubborn areas loosen up.

- Lying in bed, take long slow breaths, then start from the feet up.
- Squeeze and curl your toes for about five seconds, then release.
- Work next on your ankles, then your calf muscles, thighs, bottom; then on to your tummy (pull it in), your chest (take a deep breath), your fists, arms, shoulders, and neck (raise your shoulders to touch your ears) and even your eyelids.

Hopefully you'll be asleep before you get to the top ... but if not, just lie there and enjoy the feeling of stillness.

This technique, often called progressive muscle relaxation, has been shown in various studies to improve the sleep quality of the people who've tried it.[2]

121 ✦ Hug your other half . . .

Cuddling your loved one might not only help get you to sleep, but make you healthy all over!

Research shows hugging can reduce your blood pressure and heart rate.[3] Your body also releases the feel-good hormone oxytocin when you hug, thought to help ward off depression. Sleeping close to someone reduces the production of the stress hormone cortisol (prolonged periods of raised cortisol can trigger the inflammation that leads to heart disease). And of course, when you're less stressed, you're likely to slip into sleep mode more easily, too.

What's more, if all that hugging leads to sex, then that's great news for your sleep. Oxytocin production surges during the act, while cortisol takes a dive, relaxing you and banishing all worry. Having an orgasm releases the hormone prolactin, which also makes you sleepy. Win, win!

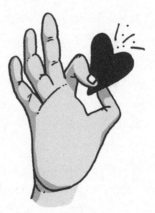

122 ✦ . . . Or do the butterfly hug!

No one to snuggle up to? No problem! Self-hugs also trigger the release of oxytocin, reduce cortisol, and calm cardiovascular stress. So fold your arms around yourself in bed if you're sleeping alone.

If you're feeling anxious, you can also try enveloping yourself in a "butterfly hug"—a method created by therapists working with children in New Mexico after they'd endured a raging hurricane.

Cross your hands and either place them on your chest or have them hugging your shoulders. Then, gently tap each alternate hand—left then right, left then right, on the chest or shoulder—like a butterfly's fluttering wings. The technique stimulates both sides of the brain and is said to help release trapped anxiety and emotions.

123 ✦ Warm your tootsies

Having warm feet could help you kick back, relax, and fall asleep faster. A study by Swiss academics published in *Nature* found that warming your feet, and thereby widening your blood vessels, helps release heat from the body's core.[4]

As we know, our core body temperature needs to fall at bedtime so as to alert our brains that it's time to sleep. So warming your toes could help nudge this natural process along and switch on the body's sleep mechanisms. One South Korean study found that people who wore socks in bed fell asleep sooner and enjoyed thirty-two minutes' more sleep with fewer awakenings than those who slept sockless.[5]

Try wearing bedsocks or toasting your tootsies on a hot-water bottle if your feet tend to feel the cold.

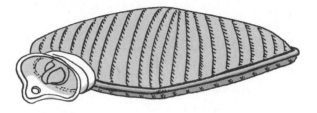

124 ✦ Melt into your bed

Imagine you're a block of chocolate or ice and that you're being gently warmed by the sun's rays and are slowly melting onto the bed.

Spread out, taking as much room as you like. Take two deep breaths, then imagine the sun warming your toes. Enjoy the feeling of the heat as it gently melts away any tension.

Moving upward, imagine the sun reaching your ankles, progressing to each part of your body all the way to your head, releasing and melting away any feelings of stiffness you're holding on to.

This is a great way to relax your muscles without needing to try too hard; and if you have particular tension in any part of your body— for example, a headache or back pain—focus on that area.

Lie still and floppy like this, as your body relaxes fully. Breathe deeply.

125 ✦ Ask for a mini back massage

A pilot study published in the *Journal of Holistic Nursing* found that patients who received a three-minute slow-stroke back massage enjoyed thirty-six minutes' more nighttime sleep than those who didn't get the treatment.[6] Massage is thought to increase serotonin, which we know the brain uses to produce the sleep hormone melatonin, and it increases delta waves in the brain, the type of waves linked with deep sleep.

Ask your partner for a mini massage before bed—just a few minutes are enough for your body to produce feelings of calm and may also bring you more shut-eye than normal.

126 ✦ Lie still

If you wake in the night, try to stay fairly motionless.

Your body interprets movements like tossing and turning as a sign that it's time to wake up, and they can trigger adrenaline production, too. So take slow breaths and focus on the softness of the sheet or duvet on your skin, or the coolness of the air on your cheek. Enjoy the stillness and the satisfaction that you're relaxing and not having to rush around.

Alternatively, working from your feet upward, focus on each body part and gently tell your mind that each one is sleepy: "My left foot is tired, my right foot is tired," and so on. If any part feels restless, try not to fight the feeling or to become anxious. Acknowledge and accept these feelings, and try to gently focus on the touch of your sheets on the restless bit before moving on with the rest of your body scan.

127 ✦ Turn that frown upside down

Being unable to sleep when you're feeling stressed is nothing to smile about, we know. But if you do smile, or even fake one, you could find it reduces your stress. University of Kansas researchers asked volunteers to hold chopsticks between their teeth in two different ways—to force the mouth either into a smile or into a neutral position—then asked them to perform stressful tasks. The heart rates of those who "smiled" recovered more quickly than their straight-faced co-participants.[7] So pretending to smile, even when you're not feeling happy, appears to lower the body's stress response.

Moving the muscles in your face into a smile also prompts a chemical reaction in the brain, releasing dopamine and serotonin, both neurotransmitters linked to feeling happy. Many psychologists believe that if we encourage ourselves to smile more through the day, then we may even be able to train our brains away from any natural tendency to think negatively and to develop a more positive mindset about everything, including our sleep.

So go on—smile, and enjoy the feelings of happiness that envelop you when you do.

128 ✦ Embrace a racing heartbeat

Through the day, unless we're heavily exercising, we rarely think about or feel our heart beating. But when we're lying in bed in the silence, we're more likely to experience a heightened awareness of it. That's all fine and dandy if you're feeling tranquil. You hear your heart beat. You ignore it. You fall asleep.

But if you're feeling anxious, hearing your heartbeat and worrying about how fast it's beating can trigger the release of adrenaline, which makes your heart beat faster and stronger. This can feel uncomfortable and make us panic. We may even think we're about to have a heart attack. All of which, of course, will banish sleep. Needless to say, if a rapid heartbeat at night is a regular occurrence, it's important to see your doctor in case it's signaling an underlying problem. But if you've gotten the all-clear, then the chances are your rapid heartbeat is simply brought on by stress and anxiety.

The trouble lies in the fact that if you experience these uncomfortable feelings in bed a few times, you begin to associate them with your bed. You lie down, fearing you're going to feel your heart beat. Stress takes over, and your heart pounds and races. It's a self-fulfilling prophecy, so don't let it become an obsession that ruins your sleep.

Many therapists advise that to feel at peace with bodily sensations you need to generate those sensations in a safe setting. It's a form of exposure therapy, designed to desensitize you to the feelings so that they don't trigger an overblown response in the form of anxiety.

To do this, run on the spot or up and down stairs for a minute, and feel your heart pounding. Stay with the feeling rather than trying to flee it. Tell yourself it's perfectly normal; it's your body's way of sending extra oxygen to your muscles.

The key is to do the exercises until your heart beating in your chest no longer produces any fear or anxiety. You may still feel your heart beat in bed, but it won't trigger a nervous reaction and send you into panic overdrive.

129 ✦ To prevent snoring, tense your tongue

If your own snoring (or your other half's snoring) is keeping you from sleeping, then doing some oropharyngeal exercises can help. Snoring happens when the soft tissues and muscles of our upper airways vibrate when they're floppy. So tightening these muscles to make them less floppy should result in less snoring!

Try pushing the tip of your tongue against the roof of your mouth behind your front teeth and then sliding it backward. Then, with the tip touching your bottom front teeth, force the back of the tongue against the floor of the mouth. Also try sucking your tongue upward against the roof of your mouth, and pressing it there.

Research from Brazil published in the American College of Chest Physicians' journal *CHEST* found that doing exercises like this resulted in a 36 percent drop in the frequency of snoring and a 59 percent drop in the level of noise.[8]

130 ✦ Try an eye mask

Various studies used to measure the sleep quality of hospital patients have found that using an eye mask resulted in better sleep and more melatonin production.[9] Not only does an eye mask help block out the light that can prevent you from making melatonin, but sometimes a gentle pressure on your eyelids can help you feel sleepier.

For an extra soporific boost, look for eye pillows that are lavender-scented.

131 ✦ Plug your ears

If you're a really light sleeper, then almost any noise can rouse you. And continual wakings mean you may complete just a couple of full sleep cycles a night. Good-quality sleep is measured by how many complete cycles we manage.

Studies have found that ear plugs can have a positive effect on hospital patients' sleep.[10] There are all sorts of plugs out there—sponge, silicon, moldable, memory foam—so you may have to experiment to see which suit you best.

132 ✦ Use a cold water bottle, or fill a sock with rice . . .

As we've discovered, overheating in bed is a common cause of sleeplessness.

If you're always searching for cool spots in the bed on a hot night, try filling one or two hot-water bottles with ice cubes instead, and place them in the bed. It's sheer bliss when your feet, arms, or legs make contact with the spots where they've been lying. It's a good idea to wrap the bottles in a thin towel in case of condensation.

Or try filling a sock with rice and pop it in a bag in the freezer for a couple of hours. It works like an ice pack or a bag of frozen peas, but without the associated sogginess as it thaws. You can place the sock onto pulse points like the back of your knees, your ankles or elbows, or lay it over your forehead for short periods.

133 ✦ . . . And chill your pillow

If it's a hot head that's stopping you from sleeping, chill your pillow. Secure it in a plastic bag and, if there's room, put it in the fridge for the day. Alternatively, just seal the pillowcase in a bag and place in the freezer. You'll get a few minutes of delicious cooling when you lie on it at bedtime, and because your neck and temples contain pulse points where blood vessels are close to the skin, it helps cool your blood down quickly so the rest of your body also feels less hot.

You can also buy cooling-gel pillows, or gel pillow mats to sleep on.

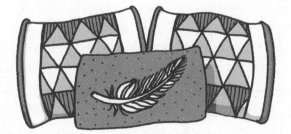

134 ✦ Flat on your back?
Try turning onto your side

If sleeping on your back is the way you sleep best and most comfort-ably, great. But a study published in *Sleep* found that poor sleepers spent most of their time on their backs.[11] This could be linked to the fact that sleeping on your back can trigger breathing problems such as sleep apnea (pauses in breathing during sleep) and snoring.

To stop yourself from sleeping this way, sew a pocket into the back of your pyjamas and place a tennis ball in it every night. Or if you have pyjamas with a pocket and they're comfy to wear back to front, do it that way. If you roll to lie on your back, the tennis ball will prod you—a not-so-gentle reminder for you to roll onto your side instead. Fixed!

135 ✦ Listen to delta binaural beats

Put on some headphones, lie back, and listen to binaural beats. These work by sending different sound frequencies to each ear, which create the illusion of a third tone; this third tone is said to influence your brain waves according to the frequency pattern used. A low frequency—or delta pattern—is associated with deep sleep. The theory is that hearing this frequency may encourage your brain waves to follow it—and be lulled to the Land of Nod.

Various scientific and medical studies have shown that listening to binaural beats can lead to better sleep, less anxiety, a reduction in cortisol, and an increase in melatonin.[12] You can buy delta binaural beat recordings, specially designed to help you sleep, online. But don't forget to wear headphones, or they won't work.

136 ✦ Soothe your eyes to sleep

Intentionally blinking lubricates your eyes and can help rest them and promote relaxation.

- Lying in bed, first relax your face by gently opening your mouth and loosening your jaw, raising and lowering your eyebrows to loosen the forehead.
- Softly exercise your eyes. Look up and inhale; look down and exhale. Look left and inhale; look right and exhale.
- Now blink rapidly about ten times, then close your eyes for twenty seconds, focusing on your breath.
- Repeat the cycle three times. Then slowly blink ten times, focusing on your deep breaths—maybe close your eyes on the inhale, and open them on the exhale.

A feeling of calm should come over you.

137 ✦ Massage your Heart 7

The "Heart 7" (also known as "spirit gate" or "mind door") is an acupressure point used to treat insomnia that might be caused by anxiety.

To locate the point (it's nowhere near your chest, by the way), go to the crease on your wrist directly beneath the point between your ring finger and your little finger. You'll feel a slight depression next to the tendon on your outer wrist. Press and hold (or lightly circle) this point for about a minute. Repeat on the opposite wrist.

You can use this trick if you wake in the middle of the night feeling anxious—or at any time of the day when you need to feel calm, as it can be done quite discreetly.

138 ✦ Stop nighttime panics in their tracks

Anxiety or panic attacks can often happen at night, as you lie there in the darkness and silence. You're going over worries you've pent up during the day? Before you know it, adrenaline starts coursing through your body, quickening your heartbeat, making your breathing shallower and your palms sweaty. Or maybe you wake up in the middle of the night with a pounding heart and a feeling of dread. Whatever the case, it's not good! The more you panic about that feeling, though, the worse it becomes.

It's certainly not easy, but you need to try to stay calm and let the feelings wash over you until they abate. Try to slow your breathing and relax your muscles. Try to take your mind to a happy place.

If lying there agitates you further, then get out of bed and walk around slowly to see if that helps, circling your shoulders to relax them. Sometimes, having a glass of cold water and swishing it around your mouth can help, or try splashing cold water over your face. This triggers the mammalian dive reflex, which slows the heart rate. (This reflex is thought to have evolved as a way to allow us to stay under water for longer—a slower heart rate means we need less oxygen.)

The main thing to remember is that your panic attack or anxiety is not going to kill you: You are not going to have a heart attack or a stroke. Accept that the effects of the adrenaline rush will probably last for about six to eight minutes. Try adopting a "Come on, let's get this over with" attitude to the whole experience.

Rather than fueling the adrenaline rush with fear, let the feelings run their course without trying to fight them. This will help you keep calm.

139 ✦ Calm your adrenals

When we encounter a perceived threat or danger, our adrenal glands (located just above our kidneys) release stress hormones, and the sympathetic nervous system is activated to help us prepare to meet the challenge and deal with the crisis. After the danger or emergency passes, our opposite, parasympathetic, nervous system is activated, allowing the body to rest up and prepare for the next challenge.

But because so many of us live under an almost constant barrage of demands, dashing around and tackling the obstacle course that is our daily routine, we're forced into a state of almost continuous high alert. Our fight-or-flight response is switched on far more than our rest-and-digest state, and our adrenals become overworked and fatigued, leading to symptoms including tiredness, the inability to concentrate, and sleep difficulties.

In reflexology, massaging the adrenal reflex on the foot is thought to help stimulate healing and calm the adrenals. You can locate the point halfway down the foot underneath the big toe at the top of the foot's arch. Press on it steadily with your thumb, using small circular motions. It may feel painful. Keep working on the area for a few minutes every day.

140 ✦ Seal off your senses

If you're struggling to relax or you feel irritable or uncomfortable, this yogic practice can help calm your mind and your nervous system.

In Sanskrit it's called *shanmukhi mudra,* "closing off the six gates"—the six gates being your two eyes, two ears, nose, and mouth. So, you're symbolically shutting off all your senses so that your mind can withdraw from all that's going on around you and focus inward instead.

You can do it sitting cross-legged on the floor before bed or when you're in bed. Raise your hands to your face, elbows pointing outward. Place your thumbs in your ears, the index fingers very lightly on your closed eyelids, lightly pressing the corners of the eyes. Put the tips of your middle fingers next to your nose, pressing the nostrils slightly without sealing them, so you can breathe through the nose quite comfortably. Your ring fingers should be placed above the mouth and little fingers below it.

Now listen to your slow, deep breathing. Concentrate on the sound as you inhale and exhale. You may see warm colors or shapes behind your eyelids. Continue for a few minutes.

141 ✦ Loosen your tongue

If trying to relax your whole body in preparation for sleep sounds too much like hard work, try relaxing your tongue, and the rest of your body might magically follow suit. Our tongues hold a lot of tension. When we're stressed, we often hold and press our tongues against the roof of the mouth without being aware of it. Check yours out now . . .

To loosen your tongue, first press it into a tense position against the roof of the mouth, then let it drop and relax. You'll probably want to let your mouth hang open as you do this. Closing your eyes, ensure your jaw is relaxed, soft, and comfortable and that both the front and back of your tongue are heavy and loose. You may begin to feel it slip backward. Swallow when you need to, then relax your tongue again.

As you concentrate on this, you may feel the rest of your body slip dreamily into relaxation, too.

The practice has a bonus advantage. Some experts say that by loosening our tongues, we loosen our minds. The theory is that when we're talking to ourselves or our "monkey mind" is chattering away in our heads, our tongues tense up, using micromovements to say the words of our inner voice. But if we relax our tongues, then our inner voices can't speak any more and so any worrying thoughts come to a halt. All of which makes it easier to slip into sleep.

142 ✦ Keep your tummy warm

The temperature of our skin is naturally higher during the night and lower during the day—that is, working in the opposite rhythm to our core body temperature, which rises during the day and drops at night.

Academics have found that very gently warming the skin (particularly the tummy area) could help you drift off to dreamland more quickly.[13] The warming increases neuronal activity in the areas of the brain involved in sleep regulation—sending a message to your body that it's time to nod off.

Try taking a *warm* hot water bottle to bed and holding it next to your belly. The key is to make sure it's not too hot, or it might have the opposite effect and make you uncomfortable, thus stopping you from falling asleep. Play around with the temperature. Just slightly warmer than your skin is the way to go.

143 ✦ Touch your lips

Your lips, especially the upper lip, are full of fine touch receptors and sensory nerve endings, meaning they're very sensitive to the touch.

It can feel comforting to touch your lips; lots of us do it through the day, to self-soothe, without even realizing it. According to the psychologist and author Dr. Rick Hanson, touching or playing with your lips may stimulate parasympathetic nerve fibers in them to switch your body into relaxation mode.[14] It may also trigger soothing emotions associated with breastfeeding.

Try lightly brushing two fingers over your lips or gently squeezing them, whichever feels more soothing.

144 ✦ Press your ear

Listen up!

It has been found that auricular acupressure—the stimulation of acupuncture points on the ear but without the use of needles—could help improve sleep. Participants in several studies have reported falling asleep more quickly plus having longer and less disturbed sleep while undergoing the therapy.[15]

The treatment works on similar principles to reflexology, according to the theory that points on the ear (rather than the foot) relate to all areas of the body. If you see a therapist for auricular acupressure they'll apply special "seeds," or magnets, to points on your ear, securing them with tape. You'll then be instructed to massage the points several times a day.

Or you can try doing it yourself.

One of the best sleep-sensitive acupressure points in the ear is the *shen men,* which is thought to relax you in preparation for sleep. Place your finger where the ear joins the head, and move it diagonally down and inward to the first dip on the cartilage part of the ear; then press and massage it or push your nail into the point for a minute.

Another area to press is the tranquilizer point, which is said to work like a shot of Valium at easing stress! It's located toward the bottom of the tragus, the part of your ear that joins the cheek.

145 ✦ The Japanese five-finger exercise

Notice how you sometimes wring your hands or clench your fingers when you feel anxious? Well, it could be that you're naturally self-soothing, and unwittingly using an ancient Japanese self-care technique called *jin shin jyutsu*. This acupressure practice involves holding on to different fingers to unblock energy flows to ease tensions. In a study published in the *Journal of Holistic Nursing*, nurses who used this technique became less stressed and enjoyed better sleep, too.[16]

The technique works on the belief that each of your fingers represents a different emotion or feeling—the thumb (worry), index finger (fear), middle finger (anger), ring finger (sadness), little finger (self-esteem). You can try this trick in bed, or any time during the day when you need to regulate your emotions!

- ✦ Start by spreading the fingers and thumb of one hand, making them long; then let them relax into a gentle curve.
- ✦ Next, using all the fingers of your opposite hand, grasp a finger or thumb, depending on which emotion you want to work on. Perhaps you're feeling angry at being unable to sleep? If so, grasp the middle finger. Maybe you're feeling stressed or worried about something? Grasp the thumb.
- ✦ Hold for two minutes. You should feel a pulse.

For extra stress-busting benefits, use your thumb to press the center of your palm.

146 ✦ Lie on your left side

Whether you're plagued by it every night or it only bothers you now and then, acid reflux or heartburn can make falling asleep seem like a distant dream. It happens when acid from your stomach leaks back up into the esophagus and causes a burning or stinging sensation in your throat and chest area. Antacids can help soothe the pain, but they can cause side effects and prove costly if you're dosing up on them daily (and nightly).

Some gastroenterology studies have shown that lying on your left side can help lessen acid reflux episodes.[17] Though experts aren't entirely sure why, it could be that this position helps keep the lower esophageal sphincter (the bundle of muscles that hold back stomach acid from entering your esophagus) above the level of the acid in your stomach.

Lying on your right side, on the other hand, may help relax the lower esophageal sphincter, making it easier for stomach acid to flow back into the esophagus. You can encourage a left-side sleeping position by placing a pillow between your legs for extra support, or hug an extra pillow in front of you.

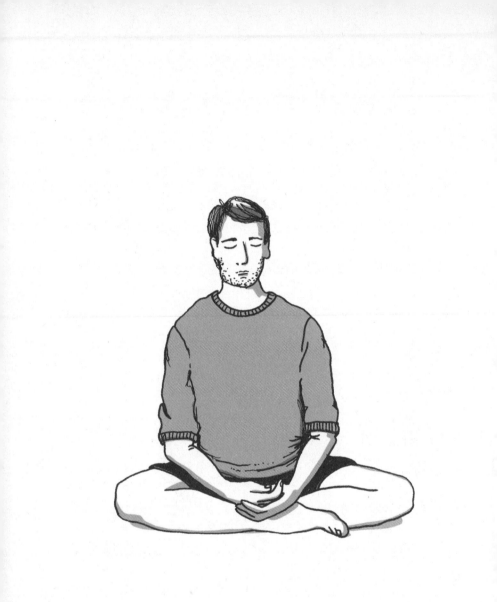

Six

Breathing Tricks

We do it all day, every day. But we barely take notice of exactly *how* we breathe. Breathing "well" and in certain ways, though, can be a big help in making you feel better both mentally and physically. Breathing techniques can engage your parasympathetic nervous system and lower your blood pressure and heart rate, all of which calms and soothes both your mind and your body.

Focusing on your breath can also make you feel more connected to your body and its well-being, and steer your mind away from worries that may be keeping you from getting a good night's sleep.

Try the following breathing tricks and exercises to help relax you into a state fit for serene sleep.

147 ✦ Do the 4-7-8 breath

Dr. Andrew Weil of the University of Arizona Center for Integrative Medicine describes this pioneering breathing technique (also called the "relaxing breath") as "a natural tranquilizer for the nervous system" because it's supposed to relax you almost instantly and help you get to sleep in minutes.

Here's how to do it:

Keep your tongue behind your upper front teeth throughout. First exhale through your mouth making a *whoosh* sound. Then close your mouth and inhale through your nose for a count of four. Hold your breath for a count of seven, then exhale through the mouth (making the *whoosh* sound again) for a count of eight.

Repeat the cycle three times and you might be ready to nod off!

148 ✦ Breathe through your left nostril

A study published in the *Journal of the Indian Academy of Clinical Medicine* found that breathing through the left nostril helped lower the heart rate and blood pressure of people with hypertension.[1]

To feel the calming effect yourself, place your right index and middle finger on your third-eye center (the space between your eyebrows), then close off your right nostril with your right thumb.

Now take long, slow, deep breaths entirely through the left nostril, aiming for six breaths a minute.

It's thought that breathing this way engages the parasympathetic nervous system, and so relaxes us.

149 ✦ Hum like a bee

This yoga technique—sometimes called "bee breath" or "humming bee"—is said to help calm you down:

Sit upright in a chair or on your bed. Gently close your eyes and mouth, keeping your teeth slightly apart.

Breathe in deeply through your nose, then breathe out through the nose, keeping your lips closed but not pursed and making a humming sound as you do so. Keep the hum going until you've finished exhaling.

You can also try bringing your hands up to the sides of your head and using your thumbs to press the cartilage at the side of each ear so as to block the ear canal, making the hum vibrate even more deeply in your head, blocking out all distractions.

Repeat five or six times and you should feel less busy-bee-like, more mellow.

150 ✦ Breathe out for longer than you breathe in

Most of us breathe too shallowly and too fast. Not only does this restrict our oxygen intake but it also relays a message to our adrenal glands that we're in fight-or-flight mode—sending our heart rate, blood pressure, and cortisol output soaring.

The 7–11 breathing technique is designed to slow everything down—breathe in for a count of 7 and out for a count of 11.

It's actually quite tough to do if you're usually a shallow breather, but you can make it easier by starting with smaller counts, perhaps breathing in for a count of four and out for six.

The important thing is to breathe out for longer than you breathe in (remember, when you breathe in your heart rate speeds up; when you breathe out it slows down). Exhaling for longer than you inhale helps stimulate the parasympathetic system, which naturally lowers your blood pressure, relaxes your muscles, and calms you.

151 ✦ Breathe like the ocean

In this breathing technique, said to calm an agitated mind and general nervousness, the aim is to make your breaths sound like an ocean wave rolling into and away from the shore.

You can do it sitting comfortably in bed or lying down.

Imagine you are trying to fog your glasses before cleaning them, making a "hah" sound but with slow, deep, even breaths. Make this long, slow sound on both the inhale and the exhale.

Practice doing it with your mouth open, and when you've mastered that variation of the technique, try it with your mouth closed. To do this you'll need to constrict the muscles by contracting the glottis (part of the larynx) in the back of your throat. In some respects this is the sort of breathing you do while asleep, so as well as calming your mind it could trick your body into sleepiness.

152 ✦ Breathe in blue

Color breathing—often used at the end of a yoga or Pilates class—involves picking a color you find calming, then breathing it in and exhaling a different color, one that represents stress. Many people find blue calming, and opt for a bright red for their exhalations, but of course feel free to choose any color that you find relaxing for this exercise.

First, start breathing slowly in through your nose for a count of 3 and exhaling through your mouth for a count of 5 or 6.

Then envision yourself enveloped in your chosen color, perhaps in the form of a cocooning blanket of light or mist. If you find it difficult to conjure up your color, picture it as the blue sky or a gently lapping blue sea.

As you inhale, imagine the calming color entering your body and filling it completely, soothing you from head to toe as it does. Now imagine you are breathing out your stress color, and envision it leaving your body along with any tension.

153 ✦ Breathe through your skin

Sometimes, deliberately trying to breathe properly to help you relax can itself cause stress. This exercise helps take the effort out of breathing, so is a good one to practice if focusing on other breathing techniques is making you feel uncomfortable or overextended.

Lying in bed, imagine that the skin all over your body is inhaling or absorbing oxygen, then expelling it. If it's easier to focus on individual parts of the body, imagine instead that the air is being absorbed through your hands or arms, then expelled through the soles of your feet. Play around with what works best for you.

Imagining this is happening should help your body relax and your breathing naturally slow down.

154 ✦ Alternate nostril breathing

Here's a novel way to use your nostrils!

It has been shown that practicing this Indian yoga breathing method regularly for six to ten weeks helped significantly reduce the heart rate and blood pressure of participants as well as reducing their stress and anxiety.[2]

Here's how to do it:

* Using your right hand, gently close your right nostril with your thumb, and breathe in through your left nostril.
* Close your left nostril with your ring finger.
* Release the thumb and slowly exhale through your right nostril.
* Now inhale through the right side, then close that nostril again with your thumb to exhale through the left.
* Repeat the sequence, until you can feel yourself relax.

You can practice this exercise first thing in the morning to give you a good start, then at night before bed or if you wake up in the night.

155 ✦ Be a square breather: Breathe yourself a box

Don't let anxiety box you in at bedtime. If you're feeling overwhelmed by thoughts and worries that are sending you into a panic, try this breathing technique. It's used by people in high-stress jobs, such as soldiers and surgeons, and aims to slow down your breathing and return it to a normal rhythm, far from fight-or-flight mode.

Start by ensuring that your tummy inflates as you breathe in and deflates as you breathe out (see "Breathe like a baby," page 136). Then breathe in for a count of four seconds as you imagine drawing the first side of a square. Now hold your breath for four seconds as you draw the next side. Next, exhale for four seconds, drawing the third line. Then hold for four seconds as you complete the final line. Erase the square on the next round of breathing, and imagine drawing it again on the following round.

Repeat several times until you start to feel relaxed.

156 ✦ Cool your body, calm your mind

If you're overheating in bed on a warm night, stress is making you feel hot and bothered, or menopausal hot flashes are bothering you, try cooling both your body and your mind with this yoga technique, called "*sitali* breath."

First stick out your tongue, then curl the sides upward to create a roll.

Now imagine your tongue is a straw, and slowly breathe in through it for a count of four or five. Then bring your tongue back into your mouth, and hold the breath for two seconds before breathing out through your nose for a count of five.

The air will feel cold as it passes through your tongue roll, cooling you down and helping calm your mind.

Some people physically can't roll their tongues, so if that's you, try this instead: Bring your top and bottom front teeth together, separating your lips. Then inhale slowly through the gaps between your teeth. Then close your mouth and exhale through your nose.

Repeat a few times.

157 ✦ Practice solar plexus breathing

Try this reflexology trick to help combat stress and the shallow breathing that accompanies it. The aim is to release tension in the solar plexus, a network of nerves in the stomach. Releasing tension here is thought to reduce pressure in the diaphragm (above the solar plexus), which can stop you from breathing deeply and filling your lungs.

◆ Sit on your bed and place your outer ankle on your knee.

◆ Squeeze the top of your foot downward and you'll see a dimpled space appear just beneath the ball of your foot in line with your second toe. This is the solar plexus point.

◆ Use your thumb to press the point firmly, inhaling as you do so.

Continue breathing as normal, but hold the pressure with your thumb for twenty to thirty seconds; then exhale slowly as you release the pressure.

◆ Repeat three times, then move on to your other foot.

You should feel your breathing becoming deeper and more free, and hopefully feel your stress melt away, too.

158 ✦ Blow bubble breaths in bed

As we all know, to blow the perfect bubble you need to take a deep breath, then blow out the bubble quite slowly and evenly or it will pop. This type of deep, slow breathing slows your heart rate and helps engage your calming parasympathetic nervous system.

Bubble breathing is a technique often employed by therapists or teachers to calm children or to treat their anxiety. But the bubble analogy can be a useful imaginative tool at any age to help exchange short, shallow bursts of breathing, typically associated with stress, for the longer, deeper breathing that can help bring calm.

Imagine you have a bubble wand. Then take a deep breath through the nose for about four seconds. Hold for two seconds; then exhale slowly through pursed lips as if blowing out a big bubble, for about seven seconds.

You can even imagine breathing "calm in, anxiety out," and envision the bubble carrying your stresses up into the air and away, until it pops and disappears.

159 ✦ **Breathe like a baby**

Lots of us tend to breathe into our chests. Check your breathing. Do your chest and shoulders move upward and outward?

This is normal during exercise or when we're tense. But a lot of us get into the habit of breathing like this all day. It can make the body feel under stress, leading to yet shallower breathing and even to over-breathing—because we feel short of breath—which can exacerbate tension and anxiety.

Babies and small children naturally breathe in the best way possible. They belly-breathe, fully saturating their lungs with oxygen while their bellies rise and fall as they inhale and exhale. This way of breathing is also called *diaphragmatic breathing* because it allows the diaphragm, the muscle that separates the chest from the abdomen, to drop down and push the belly forward so as to make room for our lungs to expand.

Not only is this kind of breathing efficient, it's also calming. It has been demonstrated that relaxed abdominal breathing can reduce our fight-or-flight response.[3]

To try belly-breathing, lie down comfortably, and place a pillow under your knees and head if that feels right. Then put something like a paperback book on your belly and a hand on your chest. The aim is for the book to move up and down as you breathe but for the hand on your chest to keep fairly still (though some movement is fine).

Breathe in and let your tummy (and the book) rise. Breathe out and allow the tummy to flatten.

If you find it difficult or a strain, don't force it. Try imagining that you're filling up a small balloon in your tummy when you breathe in and releasing the air from the balloon when you breathe out. Aim to get into the habit of abdominal breathing throughout the day and at night. Stick a note on your desk or by the fridge to remind yourself to check your breathing regularly.

The more you practice, the more natural it will become.

160 ✦ Slow it down—get to sleep sooner

Taking long, slow, deep breaths can help calm your body and your mind enough for you to get to sleep faster. Slow, regular breathing has been found to reduce blood pressure and induce feelings of calm.[4]

A study published in *Science* found the explanation as to why this might happen: it transpired that a group of neurons in the brain appear to spy on how we're breathing—and change our moods and states of mind accordingly.[5] So, by actively changing how we breathe we could change how we feel. Breathing slowly and calmly induces calm. Breathing quickly generates tension.

Most of us take about ten to twenty breaths a minute, a rate that could exacerbate stress and anxiety, so try slowing your breathing to a more leisurely six breaths a minute. Simply inhale for four seconds and exhale for six. Repeat six times and you'll have accomplished your six breaths per minute.

It may be quite difficult to slow your breathing as much as this if you're not used to it. There are some good simple apps you can use to help you concentrate on this exercise. They usually allow you to input however many breaths per minute you want to achieve, then you follow an image as it expands and contracts, matching your inhalations and exhalations to it as it does so.

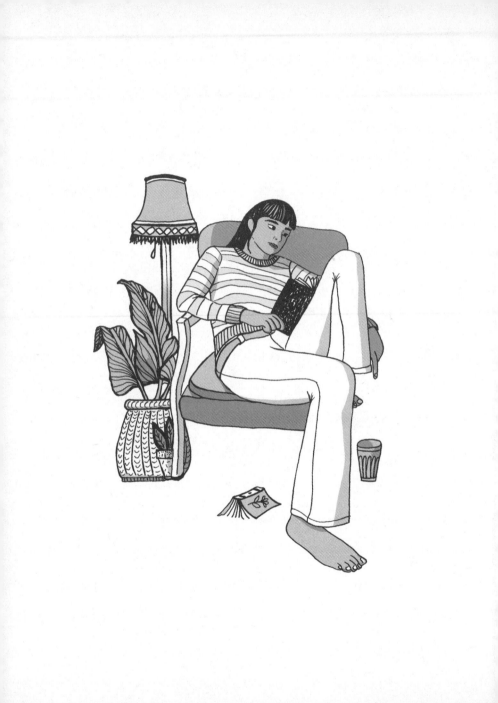

Seven

Daytime Tricks

If you spend your days on high alert, feeling stressed or anxious for a lot of the time, it's not going to be easy to get your nervous system into a calm enough state to fall asleep when your head hits the pillow. This chapter will look at healthy practices you can incorporate into your day—things to do that will help reduce your stress and teach you how to slow down and feel calmer, so that it becomes second nature to switch off when it's time for bed.

So, have a nice day … and expect a good night's sleep, too. Win, win!

161 ✦ Rise and shine

Good morning!

Getting a good night's sleep could start from the moment you wake. Open your curtains wide and expose yourself to daylight as soon as you get up. Morning light helps suppress melatonin and releases our wake-up hormone cortisol. A ten-minute dose of day-light soon after you're up will help kick-start your body's countdown to sleep, set your internal body-clock, and keep your twenty-four-hour circadian rhythm—your natural sleep–wake cycle—in check.

It works like this. If you wake and see daylight at about 7:00 AM, sleep should come naturally about sixteen hours later, at 11:00 PM. Staying cooped up in the dark (curtains closed until midday, anyone?) could delay your sleepy time until 4:00 AM, which would mean a restless night. So eat your breakfast by a window—or, even better, outside.

162 ✦ Ditch the sunglasses

To get the full benefit of the high-intensity blue wavelengths of morning light that help regulate your body's circadian rhythm, you might want to go without sunglasses for those first ten minutes of exposure when you're outside. Without shades it's easier for this light to reach the eye's photoreceptor cells, which contain a protein that transmits the signals to the brain responsible for controlling your body clock.

163 ✦ Give your brain power-breaks throughout the day

Thanks to the Internet always available at our fingertips, cell phones, and twenty-four-hour TV, we're bombarded with more information than ever. The trouble is, our brains aren't designed to pay attention for hours at a time. They can only retain full focus for about ninety minutes and then, ideally, they need to go offline for a short while to rest, renew, and recover. So give your brain little power breaks throughout the day.

Every ninety minutes or so, stop what you're concentrating on and make a cup of tea, roll your shoulders, take a short walk, or sit and simply daydream for a few minutes, or longer if you can.

By giving your brain breaks like these, you're allowing it time to process recent events and all the information it's received. Without giving it this sort of downtime, by the time you get to bed your mind will be thoroughly wired, overloaded with far too much to process to allow you to slip peacefully into slumber.

164 ✦ Turn a cup of tea into ten minutes of meditation

One way to remember to give your brain those power breaks? Switch off every time you make a cup of tea or coffee. Japanese tea ceremonies are a form of meditation, a way of finding calm and happiness in the moment. And you can perform the same sort of ritual with your own cup!

Instead of gulping it on the go, immerse yourself in the whole process. Leave your phone and tablet behind. Focus completely on the sounds of the water boiling, the steam rising, the smell of the leaves brewing. When you sit with your tea, sip it slowly and savor the taste—is it sweet or tangy, floral or fruity? How does the warm cup feel in your hand?

Completely absorbing yourself in this simple everyday act will become like a form of meditation, helping to fight frazzle, quiet your mind, and relax you. It's another instance in the day you can use to teach yourself to slow down, a skill you can exercise later in the evening when you're preparing for bed.

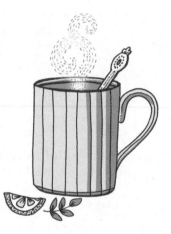

165 ✦ And eat mindfully, too

Training your brain to focus on the moment can really help when it comes to bedtime and you need to clear your mind. Practicing mindfulness like this often, throughout the day, helps you perfect the technique so it becomes second nature at lights-out. A good time to try out mindfulness is while you're eating a meal. It will feel tricky at first because, like many of us, you may be used to eating on the go, in a rush during a snatched lunch hour, or while watching television in the evening. But bear with it, and you may find you not only relax but learn to enjoy your food more, too.

First, put your phone away, turn off the TV, and sit in silence. Look at your plate and appreciate the variety of colors on it, smell the food, and feel your mouth water and your tastebuds tingle as you anticipate the flavors of what you'll be eating.

As you start your meal, close your eyes and chew slowly, really savoring the different tastes and textures—sharp or sweet, salty or nutty, and so on. Put down your fork between mouthfuls and take your time, continuing to chew thoroughly and distinguishing the different foods mingling in your mouth. This type of focus keeps you firmly in the moment.

Another bonus? Eating with such attention, without distractions, you're more likely to recognize the physical signs that you're getting full and so will be less prone to overeat.

166 ✦ Stay well hydrated

One of the main causes of waking up during the night? Mild dehydration. A dry throat can wake you, or your body could even be stirring to seek water, though you probably don't realize that's why you've woken up.

According to the Natural Hydration Council, women need about 2 liters and men about 2.5 liters of fluid a day—from water or other healthy fluids and water-rich foods like cucumber, watermelon, iceberg lettuce, celery, radish, tomatoes, green peppers, yogurts, and soups.

If you find it a struggle glugging 2 liters of water a day, try infusing it with mint, lemon, or berries for a tastier drink. Buy a large water bottle and mark it at every eight ounces, labeling each line with the hour of the day so you can be sure that you're regularly hydrating your body.

167 ✦ Schedule a problem-solving worry time

You may already have heard the advice to dump down any worries you have in a notebook before bed so you can give your mind permission to stop fretting over them and sleep peacefully. But adding potential solutions to your problems in that notepad is probably a better tactic. Psychological studies have shown that practicing "constructive worry" can help you sleep better, as it frees your mind from having to deal with things that are bothering you when you hit the sheets.[1] In essence, you're putting your worries to bed early so they don't bother you when it's your own bedtime. A study published in *Behavioral Sleep Medicine* found that volunteers asked to write down both their worries and how they might tackle them showed less "pre-sleep cognitive arousal" (in other words, repetitive worrying thoughts) than those who just jotted down their worries.[2]

Try setting aside a fifteen-minute "worry time" every evening, not too close to bedtime (say about 6:00 PM), when you concentrate on things that are troubling you.

To practice constructive worry, jot down a problem or problems that are unsettling you. Then write down a solution, or any steps you can take to resolve it. Perhaps along the lines of "I'll call Jane about that at ten AM tomorrow" or "I'll set aside time on Tuesday afternoon when I have an hour off to consider how best to tackle that difficulty." You may not have completely solved anything, but you've taken steps to—so you have things in hand.

The procedure also means your mind gets used to the concept of having a dedicated time to outpour and solve problems. So, if a worry sneaks into your mind at bedtime, threatening to sabotage your sleep, you can acknowledge it but tell yourself that you'll deal with it during worry time tomorrow.

Having your worry time somewhere other than your bed can also help break down any association you've built up between your bed and fretting. In the long run, worry time helps control how often and when you worry, meaning you will probably waste a lot less time on it.

168 ✦ Sit by a window

Being exposed to plenty of natural light during the day can help you sleep better at night. The *Journal of Clinical Sleep Medicine* published an article showing that office workers who sat next to a window slept on average forty-six minutes more at night during the working week than those who worked in offices with no windows.[3] So grab a window seat if you can. And if you can't, make sure you take your lunch outside.

Getting as much natural daylight as possible throughout the day helps your body clock stay in tune with the natural rhythms of light and dark. What's more, a daily dose of sunlight boosts our mood; lack of sunlight can make us feel depressed or anxious, which of course can also lead to sleeplessness.

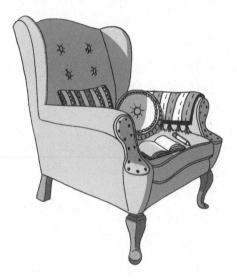

169 ✦ Don't just sit there

Commuting to work, sitting at a desk, lounging around on the sofa: statistics show that some of us are sitting, on average, a startling seven to ten hours a day. We are reliably informed that sitting for lengthy periods is linked with a whole host of health problems, including obesity and cardiovascular disease, as well as an increased risk of cancer and lower back and joint pain. What's more, staying still all day will not be conducive to sleep. You simply won't be physically tired—so move when you can.

While health experts haven't come up with an agreed limit on how long we can safely sit each day, a report commissioned by the UK Department of Health recommends that we break up our sitting time with short bouts of activity every thirty minutes.

Try setting a timer at your desk to remind you to get up and take a short walk every half hour. Make a habit of getting off the sofa during the TV ads, stand or walk around every time you take a phone call, or invest in a wearable fitness-tracker that buzzes and prompts you to move when you've been inactive for a set period.

170 ✦ Take a mindful walk

Take a break during the day to walk your way to a better night's sleep. The simple act of putting one foot in front of the other has been shown to alleviate depression, anxiety, and stress. But by making your walk "mindful" you can boost the benefits even further, according to a study published in the journal *Psychology of Sport and Exercise.*[4] Participants in the study reported lower levels of stress while walking as opposed to sitting, but found that if they walked mindfully they received even more well-being benefits.

Mindfulness is all about focusing on the present, on moment-by-moment experiences—and doing this has a calming effect. So, here's how to take a mindful walk.

As you step out, first focus on the act of walking itself, turning your attention to the physical process—your feet connecting with the ground, how your ankles, calves, and knees move.

Then expand your awareness to your surroundings—perhaps the rustle of leaves, the sound of traffic, the wind against your face, the scent of the earth. Concentrate on what you see, hear, and smell, one sense at a time. Look at everything as if you're seeing it for the first time.

In fact, walking like this is itself a form of mindfulness meditation, helping your mind find a quiet place and evoking the relaxation response. A study published in *JAMA Internal Medicine* found that twenty minutes of mindfulness meditation a day improved the sleep of adults who had trouble sleeping.[5]

This kind of contemplation break taken regularly throughout the day helps clear your head and reduces stress—and should banish those racing, sleep-unfriendly thoughts and leave you calmer, come nighttime.

171 ✦ Record a beauty spot

Next time you're taking that mindful walk somewhere picturesque, choose a pretty spot—somewhere you feel comfortable—and really focus on the scene. Use all your senses to capture the pleasant picture around you—the color of the trees and flowers, the smell of grass, the birdsong. Notice how the tranquil atmosphere makes you feel. Happy? Grateful? Calm? Content?

Next time you're lying in bed feeling stressed and unable to sleep, you can transport yourself back to this beauty spot and recall the calm and happiness you felt there, which could help you relax enough to shake off your troubles and drop off.

172 ✦ Let go of stored-up stress

Throughout the day, take regular breaks to close your eyes and check your body for where you're storing the stress. Your shoulders? Neck? Stomach? Jaw? Forehead?

◆ Breathe deeply and slowly, keeping the breath comfortable and not forced. As you inhale, imagine sending your in-breath to the area of tension. As you exhale, imagine that tension loosening like a knot in a ball of twine.

◆ Repeat for six inhalations and exhalations.

◆ If the tension is still there, gently move the area—roll the shoulders or neck, or open and close the mouth to gently release the jaw, for example.

◆ Then repeat the breathing exercise once more.

Regularly loosening up areas of tension like this during the day will help to ensure your body's not a coiled spring of tightness by the time you get to bed.

173 ✦ If you need a nap . . . take it at about 2:00 PM

Short naps can help refresh you and improve your concentration and alertness. In the past, many experts advised against nodding off in the daytime in case it compromised an individual's ability to fall asleep at night. But some now agree that if you've had a really bad night, a nap can help you make up the deficit the next day without impacting on your sleep that night.

But timing is everything. Between the hours of 1:00 and 3:00 PM we experience a small dip in core body temperature which, as we've discovered, is a signal to the brain to release melatonin, the sleep hormone. To work with this natural dip in your circadian rhythm, the ideal nap time might be around 2:00 PM.

Keep the shut-eye short, though. Ideally, your nap should last for just ten to twenty minutes and no longer than thirty. After this, you enter a deeper stage that's difficult to wake from and can leave you feeling groggy, confused, and even more tired than before. You could end up with "sleep drunkenness," which can last for up to half an hour. Napping for too long will probably interfere with your nighttime sleep, too.

Another bonus of napping? It could help retrain your brain to realize that falling asleep needn't be difficult. With no huge pressure to do so when you lie down for a nap during the daytime, the chances are you'll be relaxed and fall asleep easily.

174 ✦ Don't get caught napping on your commute

A final word on napping. Beware nap traps—when the urge to snooze can catch you unawares and impact on your nighttime slumber.

For instance, the rocking motion and white noise from a train, subway, or bus engine on your way home from work can be very conducive to falling asleep. But try not to nod off then. An early evening nap can decrease your "homeostatic sleep drive"—the body's natural urge to sleep that builds up in us steadily through the day. Think of it as having a sleep snack too late, which will spoil your appetite for sleep later that night.

If you're prone to post-work snoozing, try standing up on the commute home to keep yourself awake, or use the time to talk to a friend on the phone (if you're not in the quiet car!). Alternatively, if at all practical you could walk all or part of the way home to get some light exercise and clear your mind of work stresses, both of which can help you sleep better.

175 ✦ For better sleep, lightly exercise both your body and your brain

A study focusing on older people who had trouble sleeping found that a combination of light exercise for both the body and the brain worked better than more vigorous body and brain training.[6] Three times a week for an hour at a time, the participants were given either aerobic exercise or a gentler stretching routine to perform, along with either watching a DVD of lectures on art, history, and science or taking part in more cognitively demanding brain training sessions.

The people who reported the best improvements in their sleep were those who did the stretching exercises and watched educational DVDs.

So why not try some stretching sessions while you watch an interesting nature documentary, or call up a TED Talk on your laptop while leaning into a stretch or two, to see if it helps you get a better night's shut-eye.

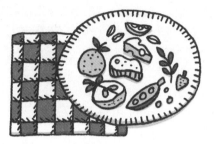

176 ✦ Boost your serotonin score

The neurotransmitter serotonin is converted into melatonin in the brain, which is why inadequate amounts of serotonin in the body have been linked to difficulty sleeping. You can try to boost your output of this chemical naturally by getting out and about in as much daylight as possible; by doing enjoyable exercise; and by eating foods said to be rich in tryptophans—which also help to produce serotonin—such as cheese, turkey, salmon, eggs, and soy products.

177 ✦ Just watch the birdies

Here's something simple we can all do to slow down during the day.

Take five minutes' time-out in your yard, go to the park for lunch, or just sit by a window at work and do some good old-fashioned bird-watching.

A study published in *BioScience* found that whether you live in a rural or an urban area, being surrounded by trees, plants, and birds can boost your mental health and bring a sense of calm.[7] The study discovered that the depth of anxiety people experienced depended on the number of birds they saw. The more birds, the less stress. And the type of feathered friends didn't matter—friendly robins, pretty blue jays, or plain old crows all boosted well-being.

You can attract birds to your garden by putting up feeders, nest boxes, and bird baths.

178 ✦ Take two-minute breathing breaks

Take little breathing breaks throughout the day to create pockets of calm that de-stress and declutter your mind so it's not overloaded at lights-out.

An easy way to do this:

- First, relax, start a timer, and work out the number of breaths (one breath equals one in and one out) you normally take in a minute.
- Once you have your figure (say, seven breaths a minute) practice a couple of mindful minutes (fourteen breaths) every so often— surreptitiously even, perhaps when you're at work and you feel a little overwhelmed.
- Settle your attention on your breath and count each in-and-out breath up to the number you calculated.
- Dab some essential oil on a tissue and breathe that in to help you focus on your breath. Choose a scent you like or one that clears your head, like eucalyptus.

Stick a Post-it Note on your computer, phone, or fridge to remind yourself to do the exercise every now and then during the day. Give yourself a breather!

179 ✦ Be more *friluftsliv* . . . and get some doses of outdoors

Natural light—outdoors—as mentioned earlier, regulates our circadian clock, our body's inbuilt way of knowing when it's time to sleep and wake. It makes us feel tired in the evening and awake in the morning.

Electric lights, TVs, and iPads, plus being indoors for large parts of the day, expose us to unnatural light patterns that confuse our body clock and can lead to trouble sleeping. So take a leaf from the Norwegians' love of heading outdoors and embracing nature, whatever the weather. Friluftsliv literally translates as "free air live."

Lots of studies have shown how being outdoors can help alleviate depression. A brisk walk or bike ride is great, but it doesn't always have to be something energetic. For instance, take an art pad into the garden and sketch some flowers, read a book on a bench in the park, or take some photos of birds and bees on a nature walk. Just spend as much time as you can outdoors so your internal body clock is clued in to what time of day it is!

180 ✦ Hold a door open, or give up your seat

Performing little acts of kindness, or perhaps volunteering at a local charity store or a community litter pick-up, not only makes you feel good but does you good, too. It's clear that helping others has an upbeat effect on the giver, making them feel happier and more positive. A study published in the journal *Annals of Behavioral Medicine* showed that people who sustain a positive outlook on life, and are generally happy, sleep better.[8]

Giving to others and being involved with people less fortunate than ourselves may also make us more grateful for what we've got. It seems that having a grateful attitude to life is linked with lower stress and a more natural ability to distract ourselves from dwelling on and catastrophizing our own problems—which, unsurprisingly, can affect how well we sleep.

If you don't have time to commit to long-term volunteering projects, do one small helpful act a day—such as letting a car in on a journey or offering to help someone with heavy bags.

181 ✦ Don't be vit-D-deficient

Vitamin D is vital for healthy bones, but it's estimated that around two in five of us is deficient. As well as vitamin D having bone-boosting benefits, research links a deficiency with poor sleep. One study of older men found that those with low levels had difficulty dropping off, and their sleep was disrupted and restless.[9] Research published in the journal *Nutritional Neuroscience* found that when twenty- to fifty-year-olds with sleep problems were given a vitamin D supplement, their sleep improved, compared with individuals given a placebo.[10]

The main source of vitamin D is sunlight and its action on our skin. Never let your skin burn in the sun. But experts say we should try to get a dose of sunlight from the end of March to the end of September, once or twice a day for ten minutes at a time and without sunscreen, to boost our vitamin D levels. According to the National Institutes of Health, some people—including older adults, breastfed infants, and those with limited sun exposure, dark skin, or certain conditions that cause fat malabsorption—may require dietary supplements to meet the daily need for vitamin D.[11]

Good sources of vitamin D are oily fish such as salmon and sardines, eggs and cereals, juices, dairy products such as yogurt and milk, and grains fortified with the vitamin.

182 ✦ Challenge unhelpful thoughts throughout the day

I've already recommended the cognitive behavioral therapy approach to challenging unhelpful and unrealistic thoughts about sleep at bedtime (see page 48, "Stop catastrophizing your sleeplessness"). But to get really good at it and so that it becomes second nature to you, it's something you need to do regularly and make part of your life. The more you practice, the easier it will be to apply at bedtime, when you need to quiet your thoughts.

So during the day, if you find uncomfortable notions are filling your head and you feel yourself becoming uptight, stop for a moment. Listen to your thoughts again. And challenge them.

It may play out like this.

First, a medley of thoughts makes you anxious: "I haven't finished that task at work; today has been awful, a complete waste of time, I'm hopeless!"

Now ask yourself if those thoughts are really true.

Might you think more realistic thoughts?

Is there a positive spin?

Rethink those thoughts.

Perhaps like this: "Yes, I probably could have managed the time better but I did complete two other tasks today, so I achieved quite a lot and I can catch up if I take a shorter lunch break tomorrow. It's not a big deal."

The key is to start to notice and appraise the thoughts that are making you anxious and unsettled.

So to recap, whenever you feel stressed, ask yourself: What am I thinking? What have I just thought? Is it a negative or unhelpful thought? Is it true? Can I look at things a different way?

Doing this practice can be a really powerful tool to stop negativity, exaggeration, or untruth from running away with you, which can increase your stress and keep you wound up like a spring all day, leaving a lot of unwinding to do when you hit the sack.

So keep practicing!

183 ✦ Try new things

Giving your brain novel experiences to make it work harder could help you sleep better. If every day is pretty much Groundhog Day and you spend it in the same environment, you're engaging only small parts of your brain. But if you give it more new opportunities, such as a trip to the seaside or a visit to a park you don't normally go to, engaging with all the new sights and sounds will help tire your grey matter—so you should sleep better at night.

In one study carried out by experts at Loughborough University people's sleep was monitored over four days—three in the lab and one experimental day when they were taken on a sightseeing tour where they experienced various new and stimulating environments.[12]

On the experimental night they felt sleepier, dropped off much faster, and enjoyed lots more deep (slow-wave) sleep, which is particularly beneficial to health. And it wasn't the physical exercise that was key to tiring them out. The same study sent a different group to a large, empty, uninspiring hall where they just walked around but expended exactly the same amount of energy as the sightseeing group. But this group didn't enjoy any sleep benefits.

So try to give your brain new experiences every day, interacting with and absorbing new surroundings. You don't have to go far out of your way. Stroll around your town like a tourist would—visit an art gallery you usually pass by, a museum or stores you never go into. Use your lunch hour to explore a park or streets you don't usually walk through. On weekends, head off to places you've never been to before.

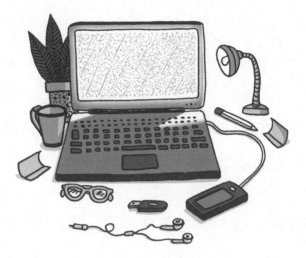

184 ✦ Leave work stress at the office

Do you breeze out of your office at the end of the day and leave all thoughts of work behind you? Then congratulations! Studies have found that being able to psychologically distance yourself from work stress when you get home means you're more likely to have a better night's sleep, and less likely to toss and turn.[13] But to rest easy you'll also need to brush off any bad feelings you've encountered during the day.

The *Journal of Occupational Health Psychology* published one study that found that people who ruminated over things that had happened at work during the day, such as coping with a rude customer, a coworker snipe, or a stern word from the boss, were more likely to sleep badly and wake several times during the night.[14]

Leaving work and its stresses behind isn't easy, of course. But there are a few steps you can take to help you relax. (Sorry, we're not talking downing vodka shots here!) The important thing is to give your mind downtime to help it recuperate from the demands of work and the strains on your mental resources. Research suggests that the following recovery experiences can help:[15]

Detach yourself from work psychologically . . .

This means you need to make distinct physical and mental boundaries between your work and nonwork life.

Imagine clocking out of work as you leave, and clocking in to your home/leisure life.

Get changed when you arrive home, for example. This can help signal to your brain that it's now "home time."

You'll also need to stop the now all too common habit of finishing off a project in the evening or answering work emails when you get home. Sometimes, we work at home out of a sense of worry or guilt. Try to stop—plenty of tasks can wait.

Relax . . .

Our bodies' nervous systems, the sympathetic and parasympathetic, work in tandem: after the stress response has switched on at work, the relaxation response should switch on when you get home. To help it on its way, take half an hour after work to do something calming: walk home for a change, instead of getting the bus; go for a leisurely swim, browse around the mall, listen to music or read a book on your commute. Schedule some relaxing things to do at home, too, if you can, even if it's just puttering in the garden.

And challenge yourself

Take part in challenging experiences and learning activities—things that help build your skills—such as playing a sport, going to an evening class, cooking a new recipe, volunteering, or even doing crossword puzzles. These sorts of activities can totally engage your mind in something other than work.

185 ✦ Say "no" more often

Stress and sleep are interconnected—that much we know. If you're highly stressed, you'll find it difficult to sleep. And if you have poor sleep, your stress can spiral. All of which means? It's pretty darned vital to try to reduce stress in your everyday life if you want great sleep.

A huge factor contributing to anxiety today is the fact that so many of us are overloaded with work and responsibilities. Most of us are simply doing too much. Our plates are piled high, and we're spinning them, too. If your deadlines and all your other obligations are weighing heavily on your mind during the day, they'll still be nagging at you at night. Expecting too much of yourself, you're always on high alert, even at bedtime.

So it's time to take action and set some boundaries.

Take a look at what you dread about your week and what you wish you didn't have to do that could free up time. Are there areas of your life you can cut back on? Are there ways you can simplify things? Are there requests from work, school, local organizations, and friends that you can say no to so that you're not overcommitting your time? The answer is usually yes. You don't have to say yes to every invitation you get. You don't have to take on extra work at the office that you simply don't have time for. You don't have to agree to help out with every community project that's happening.

Write out a not-to-do list instead of your usual to-do list, and take some pressure off yourself.

As far as possible, choose to do things that make you happy and focus on them rather than on those you do out of a sense of obligation or guilt.

Freeing up your time and your mind for some downtime of your own will help ease your stress and hopefully lead to better sleep—meaning you're well rested and so better equipped to cope with whatever new stresses life brings.

186 ✦ But do make time for your friends

Don't be a stranger! Pick up the phone and make a date to meet your friends. Numerous studies have shown the positive effects that having a supportive social circle can have on your health, including longer life expectancy. In fact, in one review of studies, which looked at the impact social connections can have on well-being, it was suggested that having a strong circle of friends can boost health as much as quitting smoking, and even more than exercising and losing weight![16] And there's yet more good news. Socializing not only makes you healthier and smile more but sleep better, too.

One study found that young people who spent more time than usual face-to-face with friends, as opposed to being on the computer or texting, fell asleep more easily.[17] Other studies, by researchers from the University of Chicago, have found not only that people who feel lonely sleep badly, but that the very fact of having sleep problems contributes to loneliness.[18]

If your schedule's looking a little sorry for itself, make an effort to mingle and book regular dates with friends, or join groups to meet like-minded people.

187 ✦ Take up a slow hobby

Knitting's not just for grandmothers and coloring's not just for kids. Relaxing hobbies like these force you to slow down and achieve what psychologists call "flow": a positive emotional state of effort-less concentration, complete focus and enjoyment—and with no stress attached.

Findings published in the *British Journal of Occupational Therapy* show that knitting can really boost your well-being.[19] Survey participants reported that the more frequently they knitted, the calmer and happier they felt. The repetitive actions of knitting can move your body and mind into an almost meditative state.

Coloring can have the same effect, helping you focus in a similar way to when you're engaged in mindfulness meditation, where your full attention is absorbed in the enjoyable task.[20] In particular, coloring reasonably complex geometric designs has been found to reduce anxiety and depressive symptoms. There are plenty of coloring books with these kinds of patterns available, and apps, too.

Other leisurely hobbies that could benefit you—and help calm an overactive mind—include doing jigsaws, gardening, and creating a mini zen garden (you can buy kits consisting of rocks and sand with which you design your own patterns). Or why not take your camera out and photograph flowers or birds?

All of these activities can help slow down your mind so it's not so wired at bedtime.

188 ✦ Stop putting things off!

Have you filed your tax return? Booked that doctor's appointment? How about calling for those insurance quotes? And what about paying your credit card bill?

If you're the sort of person who always puts things off until later, then you're up to three times more likely to suffer from sleep problems than people who keep on top of their to-do lists, according to a study by the Academic College of Tel Aviv and the University of Michigan.[21] And the more the study participants procrastinated, the worse their sleep problems. It was thought that those who put things off ruminate at bedtime about the things they haven't done, making their brains so wired and agitated that sleep seems an impossibility. This sets off a vicious cycle where procrastinators end up being too tired to complete tasks the following day—and so follows another sleepless night.

Dealing with all your tedious tasks will give you peace of mind—and peaceful sleep. So, if you're a bit of a dilly-dallier, try some of the following tips to get you motivated:

✦ Write out what needs to be done on your to-do list. Then focus on *why* each job needs to be done (for instance, I need to file my tax return or I'll get fined) and then imagine how good you'll feel after you've done it.

✦ Large tasks can seem overwhelming, so divide them into manageable chunks. So, you may give yourself the job of filling out just the first few pages of your tax return. Often, once a job is started (the most difficult part!), you'll feel encouraged and motivated enough to finish it.

✦ Set your timer for five minutes. If there are jobs on your list you think you can complete in five minutes, choose one of them and get started. Ticking it off your list could help motivate you to set the timer for another five-minute job.

✦ Reward yourself. When you've completed a dreaded task, or a chunk of it, give yourself a break and a little gift, be it a cup of coffee or a blast of your favorite music or podcast.

Your brain will come to associate completing a task with getting something good, which may become a factor in helping you fight your procrastination for good.

189 ✦ Summon up your *sisu*

We can learn a lot from our friends in Finland, who count themselves in the World Happiness Report's top five countries. According to Katja Pantzar, author of *The Finnish Way*, they're known for having a special kind of resilience—sisu—that helps them cope well with difficulties. Rather than taking a pill to solve a problem such as insomnia, for example, they're more likely to summon up their sisu, accessing their inner power to help themselves. This might mean using "movement as medicine," building as much exercise, especially incidental exercise, into their day as possible: walking, biking in all weather to and from work, and even ice-water swimming, known to boost endorphins and the feel-good hormones serotonin, dopamine, and oxytocin while reducing stress at the same time.

Sisu is also about having the determination not to give up or take the easy route—so if you can, even if it's raining outside, try bundling up and embracing all weather to get a dose of healthy outdoor exercise every day. One study found that men who exercised outdoors, walking or running, for thirty minutes fell asleep faster and had better quality sleep than those who exercised for the same amount of time indoors.[22]

So get some gym clothes that will weatherproof your workouts to see you through the seasons—and get out there come rain, snow, or wind. You'll feel—and sleep—better for it. And if ice-water swimming is asking too much, finish off your post-exercise shower with a blast of cold water instead.

190 ✦ Don't press pause on life— be sociable and active

Many people who have trouble sleeping almost put their lives on hold, canceling arrangements to meet friends and cutting back on exercise so they can try to recover lost sleep by napping during the day, sleeping in on weekends, or going to bed early at night.

But putting the brakes on your social life can actually be counter-productive to a good night's sleep. One interesting study, published in *Science*, looked at the sleeping habits of fruit flies (which, remark-ably, share much of their genetic material with humans).[23] The researchers discovered that the flies they kept in isolation slept sig-nificantly less than flies that were allowed to socialize. In the social group, the amount of sleep the flies needed rose in proportion to how many other flies they met.

The researchers surmised that as socializing is a richer and more diverse experience than being on your own, the brain needs more sleep to process it.

And while it's understandable that running low on sleep might make you less motivated to lace up your sneakers for a 10K run, it's still important to keep active and moving.

A study found that sedentary adults suffering from insomnia who were prescribed aerobic activity improved their sleep significantly compared to other poor sleepers who didn't exercise.[24] They also reported having more energy and feeling less depressed.

Remember, a healthy life is all about balance. So as well as finding time to relax and rest, do keep active, and don't cancel that dinner date with your friends. The key is to fill your life with pleasant experiences so that sleep and insomnia don't become the main focus of it. In the long run, having a rich and fulfilling life should do the trick.

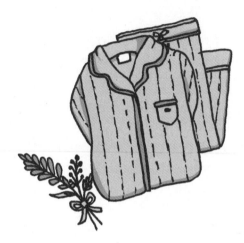

191 ✦ Schedule some pamper time

As we've seen, being stressed has been widely and authoritatively linked with insomnia, and being unable to sleep with exacerbating stress. Whichever came first, the stress or the sleeplessness, one thing's certain: getting back some serenity in your life can only help you sleep better at night.

You may have heard the term "self-care" being tossed around a lot lately. It's nothing new—just a new way of saying "Take better care of yourself." At its simplest, self-care is about making sure you eat healthily and get enough exercise, but to boost self-care's stress-busting benefits it's important to give yourself the time and space to relax, especially if you're the sort of person who usually (always?) puts other people's needs first. When you're continually caught up in caring for others, seeing to and anticipating their needs and wants, you're often on high alert or at the very least depriving both your mind and your body of the chance of some much-needed downtime. And if you're on high alert when you hit the hay? Needless to say, you'll struggle to nod off.

In short? It's important to pamper yourself from time to time.

For you, that might mean a scented bubble bath, listening to music, or relaxing with a good book. Or it might mean meeting friends for coffee, cooking a favorite meal, taking to two wheels on a bike path, visiting an art gallery, or doing some yoga.

Schedule in time for when you'll do some of your pampering. This is important, or chances are it just won't get done.

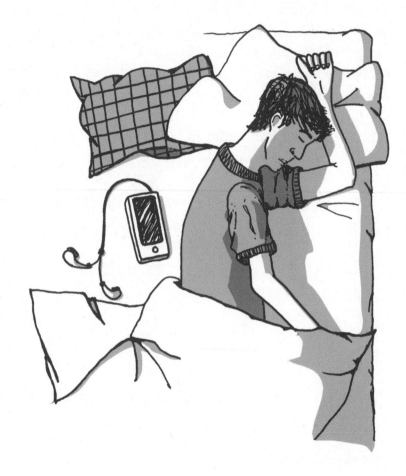

Eight

Tips for Taking the Stress Out of Sleep

This chapter will equip you with super sleep knowledge, so you know what can help—and hinder—your chances of enjoying deep, reassuring shut-eye. Understanding more about slumber will mean you can work with your body and your mind's natural ability to nod off. No problem.

It's packed with tricks and techniques you can incorporate into your everyday life: treatments to try, self-help remedies, and mindset manipulations that should have you looking at sleep in a better light. All of which adds up to less stress and more serenity, when you lie down at lights-out.

Learn to fall in love with falling asleep again.

192 ✦ What's your chronotype?

Are you a night owl or an early bird, or do you fall somewhere in between? Knowing which type you are could be the key to a better bedtime.

If you're naturally an owl, going to bed too early could mean you lie there for hours struggling to nod off. You feel frustrated, and you may begin to think of your bed as a place of wakefulness rather than sleepiness. Here's what to do to find out your chronotype—your individual natural sleep and wake times.

Next time you're on a break, away from your normal routine—ideally for a week or longer—hit the hay only when you feel really sleepy and get up when you wake naturally, without an alarm.

After you've discovered your body clock's rhythm, when your ideal bedtime is and how much sleep you ideally need, you can stick to this new pattern at home, or at least aim for as close to it as possible, depending on your commitments. Bear in mind that not everyone thrives on the ideal eight hours; some need more, others less.

Discovering your body clock's personal preference means you can work *with* your chronotype, rather than against it.

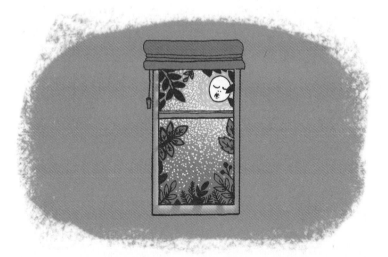

193 ✦ Make friends with your feelings and welcome unwelcome thoughts

Lying in bed awake with no distractions means you can often become acutely aware of what you wouldn't notice in the daytime when you're busy. We've already discovered that your heartbeat can seem loud or fast; worries can flood your mind and whirl around in overdrive. It's natural to tense up against unwelcome thoughts and feelings, to try to flee from them or push them away. But this sends a message to your body to pump out adrenaline, forcing you into fight-or-flight mode, which in turn makes that rapid heartbeat faster and those thoughts more panicky. A vicious cycle of anxiety!

Instead, accept the thoughts calmly, and by doing so give your body and your brain a different message.

The sleep specialist Dr. Guy Meadows, a proponent of acceptance and commitment therapy for insomnia, suggests an unusual response to unwanted thoughts and feelings. Instead of trying to push them away, he says, welcome them as you would a friend. Even say something like "Oh hello, anxiety—you again?" or "Welcome back, worry," in a lighthearted way. Just this simple action can help you become more physically and mentally relaxed because you're informing your brain that you are safe, not under any threat.

Once the welcome is made, you can turn your attention to something pleasant, such as enjoying the sense of relaxation as you lie down, or the warmth from your duvet.

194 ✦ Chillaxercise!

Exercise that increases your heart rate is great for cardiovascular health, and if you also incorporate a slow exercise into your week you'll get a host of other health benefits, too.

Disciplines like tai chi, qigong, and yoga not only offer physical gains such as improved flexibility, balance, and strength, but they also teach you how to be comfortable with slowing down, retraining your body and mind to find calm and to be better able to cope with stress.

Don't think you have to be expert at them, either. Join a beginners' class or just watch a video online and try it out. You may well find you sleep better.

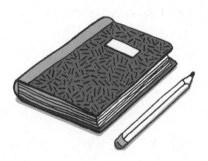

195 ✦ Keep a sleep journal

Filling out a journal can help you track any patterns that may be leading to poor sleep.

Buy a large notebook that appeals to you and that you'll enjoy using. Look online for "sleep journal" templates you can copy into it.

◆ Mark out opposite pages in your notebook with seven columns for the days of the week—the left page to fill out every morning, the right to fill in every evening before bed.

◆ On the first left-hand page, add sections in the margins to fill in each morning, including the time you went to bed and got up; how long it took you to fall asleep; how many times you woke in the night; what you think woke you (stress, noise, discomfort?); and how you felt at the start of the day (refreshed, groggy?).

◆ On the opposite, evening, page, add sections where you can fill in what you ate and drank and when, including how late you had your last caffeinated drink and last food; what kind of day you had (stressful? relaxed?) and what you did; how long you exercised for, and when; any naps you took; and what you did in the last hour before bed.

◆ At the end of each week, examine your journal for any patterns that might have emerged and see if you can evaluate whether any of your actions seem to be helping or hindering your sleep. What did you (or didn't you) do on days you slept well? What had happened during the day on nights you slept badly?

Your journal may reveal, say, that you sleep badly on Friday nights (after too much alcohol, for instance?) or on Wednesdays after your 9:00 PM spin class (maybe you're exercising too late in the evening?). Identifying patterns could help you take steps to change your habits to improve your sleep.

Don't feel overwhelmed. Concentrate on changing one habit at a time, and you could soon be on the road to solving some of your sleep problems.

196 ✦ Enjoy comedy!

Giggling more during the day could help get you to sleep.

A study published in the Korean *Journal of Adult Nursing* found that elderly people who were prescribed laughter therapy, which included singing funny songs and laughing exercises, improved their sleep and reduced their symptoms of depression.[1] Another, Japanese, study discovered that nursing mothers who had watched a comedy DVD had more of the sleep hormone melatonin in their breast milk than those who had endured an unfunny weather news DVD.[2]

So you may want to watch more comedy instead of dramas (or weather reports!) to get a good night's sleep.

197 ✦ To reset your body clock, try camping!

If you're thinking of taking a break, consider camping.

Researchers from the University of Colorado found that a group who spent a week sleeping outside in tents, with no manmade light allowed (only natural light and campfires), nodded off more easily and woke more refreshed than usual.[3]

Exposure to a natural light–dark cycle helped their melatonin levels rise earlier and synchronize their internal body clocks to natural, healthy sleep rhythms.

Our bodies respond quite quickly to nature's light–dark cycle, so spending plenty of time in natural daylight and filling the nights with more true darkness for a weekend of camping, or even just being outdoors through the day and evening, should be enough to have an impact on your circadian rhythm and promote better sleep.

198 ✦ Learn to elicit your relaxation response

Coined by the cardiologist Dr. Herbert Benson, the term "relaxation response" is defined as your ability to switch your body into a calm state—slowing your heart and breathing rates, lowering your blood pressure, and clearing cortisol from the body.

In essence, it's the opposite of the fight-or-flight (or stress) response. You can learn how to elicit your relaxation response, tapping into a resource within you, to conjure up calm. The technique involves using a gentle word or phrase, or a prayer, and repeating it.

- First, think of the word you'll use: something like "peace," "calm," or "love."
- Sit still and close your eyes. Breathe slowly and, on each out-breath, silently say your chosen word. If other thoughts or worries enter your head, don't be upset by them, just say "Oh well" in your mind and resume your repetition.
- Continue for five to ten minutes and don't worry if you're bombarded by everyday thoughts and are mostly saying "Oh well," or similar.

Keep practicing the technique (every morning before breakfast is good, but any time of the day will do), and with time you'll find it easier to focus on your breath and your chosen word. The more you practice, the better able you will be to evoke the relaxation response at night if you need it.

199 ✦ Find your *ikigai*

The Japanese word "ikigai" is often translated as "having a purpose in life" or "what makes life worth living." Your ikigai could be anything from your children, or a hobby you can't get enough of, to your job. And as well as giving your life meaning, it seems that having a strong sense of ikigai could also be key to sleeping more soundly.

A study published in the American journal *Sleep Science and Practice* in 2017 found that people who have a strong life purpose were more likely than others to enjoy good quality sleep.[4]

Can you name your ikigai? If not, then it may be worth taking time to find a new purpose in life. Think about volunteering to help others. Or taking up a hobby you've left behind, or a new sport you've always wanted to try.

It could be that this passion and purpose becomes the thing that gets you out of bed in the morning and also helps you sleep at night.

200 ✦ Restrict your sleep

It may sound counterproductive, but try this experiment—go to bed later than normal and spend less time there. It could help you get lengthier and better sleep in the long run. One study found that this practice, called *sleep restriction*, helped people with insomnia fall asleep sooner and stay asleep for longer when they tried it over a period of eight weeks.[5] So it's not achieved overnight and will require commitment. Here's how to do it if you want to try it out:

Using a sleep journal (see page 174), calculate how much time you spend in bed and how much of that time is spent awake. If you're spending less than 80 percent of your total time asleep, you're probably lying there for too long—and you're learning to associate your bed with sleeplessness.

So, consulting your sleep journal, if you're getting an average of, say, six hours a night over the course of a week and you normally need to get up at 6:00 AM, hold off going to bed until midnight, even if you feel sleepy before then. The aim is to build up your "sleep pressure" so that you fall asleep quickly when you go to bed, and get a more solid night's sleep, too.

This practice could help you regain confidence in your ability to nod off soon after your head hits the pillow and keep blissfully sleeping until it's time to get up.

Keeping track in your journal, when you've found that for five or six days you're sleeping for most of the six hours you're in bed, go to bed fifteen minutes earlier. Keep up this pattern and hopefully you'll be able to consolidate a better one, with longer and better sleep.

Plus you'll boost your sleep confidence—and fall in love with your bed again.

201 ✦ Do yoga daily

Whether you prefer downward dog or camel pose, yoga moves could help you get better z's. The stretches can help calm your nervous system whenever you're feeling overstimulated or stressed. A Harvard Medical School study found that insomniacs who were taught yoga and practiced it every day for eight weeks improved their sleep quality, dropping off more quickly and staying asleep for longer.[6]

Join a local class or learn at home from a DVD or YouTube videos online. Remember, you don't have to be an expert or wonderfully flexible to get the benefits of yoga.

Doing it daily seems to provide the best benefits, so try to incorporate a few yoga poses and breathing exercises every morning or after work.

202 ✦ Stay regular, but don't obsess about it

Our bodies like routine, so sticking to a regular sleep schedule, like we did as little kids, could help synchronize our sleep-wake cycle and strengthen our bodies' circadian rhythms. This means going to bed at the same time every night and waking up the same time every morning, even on weekends or after you've had a bad night and the temptation is to sleep in.

With good routines, your body gets to know exactly when it should be releasing your sleep and wake hormones. If you keep changing your bedtimes and wake times, or sleep in for hours on the weekend, you may well send confusing messages to your inner body clock.

Of course, you don't need to keep to a completely tight schedule—we all have busy lives when sometimes it's just impossible to get to bed on time or wake on time in the morning. So the caveat is this: worrying unduly about being late to bed and sticking to a strict schedule will just stress you out. And that's not conducive to falling asleep quickly.

But if you can try to keep to within an hour of your regular times, the payoff could be better sleep.

203 ✦ Get enough exercise

If there's one thing we should all be doing to improve our overall health it's getting plenty of exercise. Not only can it boost our cardiovascular health, help lower blood pressure, and tackle obesity, but numerous studies have shown that being active, whether you're a young adult or a retiree, can have a big effect on how well you sleep.[7]

It's clear that taking part in regular exercise can help us drop off, increase how long we sleep, help us get more restorative sleep, and wake less during the night. It doesn't seem to matter what type of exercise you do—aerobic or a mixture of aerobic and resistance training. The key seems to be to make it a regular habit, as well as to reach at least the current recommended guidelines for physical activity. This means aiming to be active every day, and that over a week we should be doing at least 150 minutes of moderate-intensity exercise such as biking or brisk walking, in bouts of 10 minutes or more; or 75 minutes of vigorous-intensity activity spread across the week; or combinations of the two. Examples of vigorous activities are running and playing sports like soccer.

Health guidelines also say we should be doing muscle-strength-training exercises, such as lifting weights, at least two days a week.

Your body temperature stays elevated for a few hours after exercise. As your core temperature needs to drop in order for you to fall asleep easily, it's best, if you can, to avoid anything but light exercise such as gentle stretching, restorative yoga, or a leisurely walk within a couple of hours of bedtime.

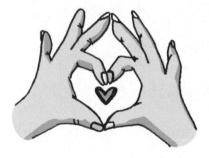

204 ✦ Be kind to yourself when you can't sleep

If you're lying awake at night feeling frustrated and angry with yourself for being unable to nod off, try treating your struggling mind and body with kindness instead.

By soothing ourselves we trigger the release of oxytocin, which can help us feel calm. Research also shows that feeling cared for can lead to less stress. In one study people were asked to imagine receiving compassion from someone.[8] They were verbally prompted every sixty seconds with statements such as "Allow yourself to feel that you are the recipient of great compassion," or "Allow yourself to feel the loving-kindness that is there for you." The result? Afterward, the participants were found to have lower levels of cortisol, a hormone that will surely stop you from sleeping.

When we're being self-critical, on the other hand, our bodies see it as an attack of sorts, and go into fight-or-flight mode, leaving us feeling tense and edgy.

Start by listening carefully to how your body and mind are feeling. Notice any tension or anxiety but don't fight it or try to fix it. Instead—though you may feel a little silly at first—try tenderly stroking your arm or face, or gently tap your body as you'd try to comfort a baby or small child who was struggling to sleep.

Talk soothingly to yourself. Use phrases like "Be calm, be peaceful. You've had a long day. Relax now." Showing yourself compassion can switch off your stress response and trigger the relaxation response instead.

There, there.

205 ✦ Go forest bathing

Shinrin-yoku is a Japanese term meaning to immerse yourself in the atmosphere of the forest. This practice of forest bathing—walking slowly through woods and forests, watching nature and inhaling the trees' essential oils—has been found to offer a host of physiological and psychological health benefits. These include helping to lower stress, to boost the immune system, and to improve people's mood.

And it seems trees could also help you get better sleep. A Japanese study revealed that wandering through woods improved the depth and quality of the participants' sleep.[9]

If you have countryside, woods, or forests near you, spend time exploring them and walking mindfully through them, using all of your senses to soak up the atmosphere around you.

206 ✦ Or bring the forest indoors

If you can't go down to the woods today or you live in the middle of a city, try bringing the forest indoors—it can offer the same benefits.

Use essential oils from trees such as eucalyptus, Douglas fir, or cedarwood to scent your home in oil burners or diffusers. Bring plants into your house and workplace. Studies have shown that just looking at foliage plants, roses, and bonsai trees can reduce stress levels and relax the body and mind.[10]

207 ✦ You can bounce back

If you've had a couple of sleepless nights, it can set off a vicious circle of sleeplessness. Why? Because if you start to worry—panic, even—about what the lack of sleep is doing to your health, how you're going to cope at work, how tired you're going to look, how on earth you're going to function generally . . . and so on, and on, and on . . . your brain can't switch off and let you sleep . . . leading to more and more sleepless nights.

But the good news is that you *can* bounce back from a couple of bad nights. Scientists have discovered that the body has its own clever recovery system that helps make up for small periods of lost sleep, by spending more time in the deep sleep stages once we do fall asleep—the kind that restore us both physically and mentally—and less in the lighter stages.

So you can make up for the sleep debt of a couple of wakeful nights over the next two nights. Armed with this knowledge, don't let worry keep you awake!

208 ✦ Try autogenic training

This relaxation method can teach you how to calm your nervous system and even gain some measure of control over your heart rate, blood pressure, and breathing. You can sign up for a course, or there are apps to help you learn the technique.

A study carried out by the Royal London Hospital for Integrated Medicine found that people who underwent an eight-week autogenic training course fell asleep more quickly at bedtime as well as if they woke during the night.[11] Plus, they felt more energized and refreshed when they woke up.

This method, a form of self-hypnosis, works on the premise that relaxation can be induced by suggestion. You learn to focus awareness on different parts of the body, then nurture sensations of warmth, tiredness, or heaviness—for instance, by repeating to yourself a script containing lines like "My right arm is heavy, my left arm is heavy, my arms are heavy." "My right foot is warm, my left foot is warm, my feet are pleasantly warm." "My heartbeat is calm and regular."

In some ways it's like a verbal body scan. You can practice the exercises a few times a day and during your bedtime wind-down routine.

209 ✦ Do a tech detox

It's become the norm to respond to texts and tweets in seconds—with some of us swiping and checking our phones a staggering 2,617 times in one day. But using tech nonstop like this can make us cranky and keep our brains wired so that we find it hard to wind down at bedtime. Some experts are already advising that excessive use of tech and social media should come with a health warning, many of them suggesting it's more addictive than cigarettes and alcohol.

Numerous studies have found that the pressure to keep up to the minute with updating social networking sites results in a great deal of tension and anxiety. When a study from the University of Copenhagen asked regular Facebook users to take a break from the site for a week, they reported better life satisfaction, feeling happier and less stressed.[12] Researchers at the University of California found office workers who checked their emails frequently had elevated "high-alert" heart rates, while those who took a five-day break from email experienced more natural, variable heart rates, a sign of good health.[13]

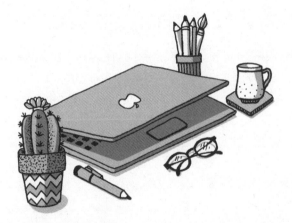

Being in a state of high alert throughout the day is just not conducive to sleeping well, as we have seen. So make an effort to take tech breaks—not just at night but throughout the day, too. If you're a tech addict, at first try putting your phone away for short periods—while watching TV or walking the dog, for example. Extend the amount of time you go between picking it up. Turn off notifications or at least tweak what you receive, so that your phone isn't constantly tempting you to take a look at Facebook or Twitter likes, app updates, or incoming email.

Ironically, there are apps that can help you detox from tech. The Forest app, for example, lets you plant a seedling and "grow" a tree, which will die if you use your phone for anything other than necessities like taking calls. Plus, you receive credits to use to plant real trees around the world, thus enabling you to play your part in helping the environment.

210 ✦ Check your meds

Lots of commonly prescribed pills, such as alpha-blockers and beta-blockers (used to combat high blood pressure), SSRIs (selective serotonin-reuptake inhibitors) for depression, and corticosteroids used to treat inflammation and rheumatoid arthritis, have been shown to disturb sleep in some people. Some over-the-counter medicines such as pain-relief or cold and flu treatments can contain caffeine, and ingredients in decongestants can mimic the effects of adrenaline, causing nervousness, a fast heartbeat, and insomnia.

If you think that your medication may be affecting your ability to sleep well, read the accompanying leaflet thoroughly and talk with your doctor or pharmacist about looking at any alternatives or about changing the time of day you take your pills.

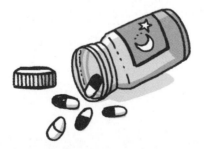

211 ✦ Don't fear waking during the night—it's normal

If you wake up with an "Oh no, not again, why me?!" attitude, immediately anxious that you won't be able to fall back to sleep—then you probably won't. It becomes a self-fulfilling prophecy, and often one that subsequently happens night after night.

But what if you knew that waking up several times a night is absolutely normal and that it happens to everyone, so it's really no big deal?

We sleep in cycles averaging about ninety minutes each. As we reach the end of one cycle, we may wake for a short period before slipping quite seamlessly into the next one. Regular stirrings may possibly hark back to when we were cavemen and we'd wake periodically to scan for predators. They also give us a chance to change position, of course, so we don't get sore points or dead arms. Good sleepers might not even notice that they've woken, or they just turn over and immediately fall back to sleep. Problems start when you realize you've woken, then get anxious about being unable to nod off again.

When you do wake like this, try not to feel frustrated. Instead, accept it as a normal part of your sleep cycle. Smile, breathe deeply, and enjoy the fact that you're lying in bed and that it's not yet time to get up.

Recognizing that waking is a normal part of the night should make you more relaxed about it and help you drop off again quickly.

212 ✦ Clear the air

It has been found that people who live in areas with high air pollution can be up to 60 percent more likely to sleep poorly than those who live in areas with cleaner air.[14] It could be that the pollution causes irritation in our noses and throats, which can affect sleep, or even that very small particles can get into the bloodstream and affect the regulation of sleep in the brain.

Try using an air purifier to clean the air in your home. Some have built-in sensors that switch on the appliance when the air quality drops—for example, if there's a build-up of traffic outside.

If you are using one in your bedroom, make sure you choose a quiet model. Some come with a special night-mode setting designed not to disturb your sleep.

213 ✦ Get needled

Studies suggest that acupuncture can be an effective treatment for insomnia, concluding that individuals who had acupuncture sessions fell asleep faster and experienced a better quality of sleep than those who had sham acupuncture or a placebo.[15]

This ancient Chinese medicine uses needles to stimulate pressure points on the body to influence the nervous system and relieve stress and tension. It's also thought to increase the body's nighttime secretion of melatonin, the sleep hormone.

Do find a reputable, qualified practitioner—ask for recommendations and visit the website of the National Certification Commission for Acupuncture and Oriental Medicine (NCCAOM), the US's main regulatory body for the practice. Don't expect a quick fix, though. Most studies have shown that treatment involves at least five weeks of regular sessions to see effects on sleep.

214 ✦ Stop smoking

It's as simple as that, I'm afraid. Puffing is not only linked to lung cancer and heart disease: research has shown it could turn you into a poor sleeper, too.[16] Nicotine is a stimulant, so smoking too close to bedtime can stop you from nodding off. In addition, dependency can cause sufferers to wake in the night because of withdrawal symptoms.

Breathing difficulties among smokers can also make for restless nights. A study from the University of Nebraska Medical Center found that smokers were two and a half times more likely to have obstructive sleep apnea—where the airway becomes totally blocked for ten seconds or more—than non- and former smokers.[17]

To try to quit, visit betobaccofree.gov or get in touch with Quitline: 1-800-QUIT-NOW (1-800-784-8669), a free telephone support service that helps people who want to stop smoking. Calls are diverted to your own state Quitline, which offers advice, practical information, counseling, and ways to cope with nicotine withdrawal as well as free or discounted medications to help in some instances.

215 ✦ Don't fight for more sleep than you need

Getting eight hours' sleep a night might seem to be the Holy Grail when it comes to recommendations for optimum amounts. But do we all really need that much? It's been a contentious issue among sleep scientists, but most would now agree that just as we all need to eat differing amounts of calories to keep a steady weight, so we all have different sleep needs.

Your personal ideal sleep quota can depend on everything from your genetics to how active you are and your general health. While some of us thrive on eight hours, others get by on six and a half. The key is there's no need to obsess about how much sleep you're getting if you don't feel excessively sleepy during the daytime. Remember, we all get dips and troughs in how alert we are through the day, no matter how much sleep we get.

So the message is this: if you're heavily focusing on (and fretting about) achieving a solid eight hours a night, then you're creating unnecessary stress that could, ultimately, stop you from sleeping!

Think about setting yourself lesser goals and instead, focus on getting good quality rest. If you relax more about exactly how much sleep you're getting, you never know, you may just achieve more sleep anyway.

216 ✦ Get some vitamin sea

Take a trip to the coast whenever you can! Not only has research found that people living within a half mile of the sea generally feel healthier than those living further away,[18] but a report by the UK National Trust found that people who took a coastal walk slept on average forty-seven minutes longer that night than they did the night before, and thirty-five minutes longer than people who took a walk inland.[19]

Some experts say that listening to ocean waves has a calming effect and that it changes the frequency of our own brain waves, putting us into a mildly meditative state. It's also thought that our brains hear the ocean, with its gentle and gradual variations in volume, as a nonthreatening noise, something we can almost ignore or zone out, but which at the same time activates the parasympathetic nervous system, slowing our heartbeat and relaxing us.

If you can't get to the beach, listen to an app or a download of ocean-wave sounds at bedtime.

217 ✦ Time your bedtime perfectly

As noted earlier, we sleep in cycles of about ninety minutes, going from wakefulness to light sleep to deep sleep to REM—rapid eye movement, when the brain is active and dreams occur—then back again in continuous loops. The quality of sleep is measured by how many complete cycles we manage.

If you want to maximize the number of cycles you get and to wake up feeling refreshed and ready to take on the day (and who doesn't?), you should aim to wake every morning at the end of a sleep cycle when you're naturally close to wakefulness, rather than in midcycle when you're in deep, restorative sleep.

To increase your chances of waking up at the end of a cycle, do this quick calculation:

Decide on the time you need to be awake—say 7:00 AM—then count backward in blocks of ninety minutes: 7:00 AM; 5:30; 4:00 AM; 2:30; 1:00 AM; 11:30 PM; 10:00 PM. So you need to try to fall asleep around 10:00 or 11:30 PM to complete either five or six sleep cycles and wake up ready and raring to go!

Head off to bed about twenty minutes before your ideal sleep time.

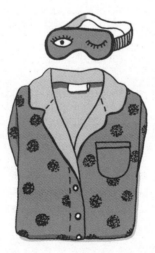

218 ✦ How to beat jet lag, and sleep

Our body's circadian rhythms can go loopy after crossing time zones on long-haul flights. When you get to your destination you'll either feel sleepy when everyone else is enjoying their afternoon, or wide awake when everyone else is fast asleep. Try these tips to help you adjust and sleep like the locals:

✦ Before you fly, take a few days to try to shift your body clock in line with where you're going. Go to bed and get up earlier if flying east, and later if flying west.

✦ As soon as you take off, adjust your watch to the time it is wherever you're heading. If it's already bedtime there, try to sleep—use an eye mask and ear plugs to create nighttime. If it's morning over there, put on your night light and try to stay awake.

✦ On arrival, to reset your body clock at your destination, try to get out and about into sunlight (an early morning walk is especially good).

219 ✦ To sleep soundly you must feel safe

You need to feel safe at night to sleep well. Any fears you may have about being robbed or having a fire in the house, for example—or even after watching a scary film or the news—could keep you in a state of high alert and interfere with your sleep.

So if you hear a movement or a creak that you can't identify, your body's sympathetic nervous system will activate your fight-or-flight response. This will release adrenaline, which ramps up your heart rate and blood pressure, making it difficult to switch off and sleep. If you do drop off, chances are you'll still be in a state of hyperarousal, with your brain (and subconscious mind) more active than it should be, monitoring what's going on around you. So sleep will be light, not refreshing, and you'll easily be woken.

Take action to feel safer. This might mean getting a house alarm fitted and using it at night, checking smoke and carbon monoxide alarms are working, installing better door and window locks. It may also mean, if you find the news is disturbing you, that you take a break from watching or listening to any updates after 6:00 PM. And avoid horror films, true-life crime stories, and disturbing books before bed.

If you do suffer from fear or anxiety at night generally, then try to make your evenings calm and carefree—watch some comedy or a lighthearted film, or read a book that won't put you on edge at lights-out.

220 ✦ Forget rose-tinted glasses, go amber

So, we know that the blue light emitted by our smartphones, tablets, and laptops can keep us awake by suppressing melatonin production, but most of these devices have nighttime settings that emit amber instead of blue light to combat this problem. What, though, about the blue light that comes from our televisions, computers, and LEDs? The answer could lie in putting on a pair of amber-tinted glasses.

Researchers from Columbia University asked a group of people diagnosed with insomnia to wear amber-tinted glasses for seven nights in the two hours before bedtime.[20] Four weeks later, they were instructed to wear placebo clear glasses for another seven nights. It turned out that they had on average around thirty minutes' longer and sounder sleep on the nights they'd worn the amber lenses.

Ask your optician about amber-tinted lenses, or search online.

221 ✦ Be more optimistic

While not getting enough sleep may make you grumpy and pessimistic, there's a plethora of research out there that indicates being a pessimist could itself make you a poor sleeper.[21] People with a negative outlook on life are generally more anxious and suffer more symptoms of stress, which we know can adversely affect sleep. For example, pessimists are more likely to lie in bed thinking about what could go wrong with their sleep tonight, rather than what could go right!

Optimistic people not only enjoy better sleep, but studies have shown they have better heart health and are more likely to live longer, too.[22] But can you make yourself more optimistic? Yes, say psychologists, you can learn to adopt a more upbeat outlook. Try the following two tips:

Positive reframing

Next time you have a bad day take time to write down anything about it that was positive. Perhaps your car broke down. You moaned about it on Facebook and a friend you hadn't spoken to in a while sent a message. She asked to meet up and you've set a date. Result! Your partner realized how stressed you were after having to wait around for a tow truck and cooked you your favorite meal to make you feel better. Not a bad day, after all?

Regularly practicing positive reframing like this can help train your brain to find the positives more often, without prompting, helping you cultivate a more automatically optimistic frame of mind.

Mix with positive people

Pessimistic people give off negative vibes, whereas optimistic people emanate positivity—and both can be contagious. If you spend too much time with people who complain or snipe, it rubs off on you. Similarly, being surrounded by happy individuals means you're more likely to be cheerful, too, as research has shown.[23] So surround yourself with as many positive people as you can.

222 ✦ Oils are essential!

Aromatherapy—inhaling essential oils extracted from aromatic plants—is believed to have a therapeutic effect on our brains and bodies, and has been shown in several studies to help calm the mind, relieve stress, and make it easier to drift off to dreamland.[24]

You can use aromatherapy oils in lots of different ways. Add them to your evening bath, dot onto pot pourri in the bedroom, warm them in a diffuser, mix with water and spritz onto your pillow, or add them to carrier oils and massage into your skin. Oils thought to have soporific and calming qualities include lavender, jasmine, geranium, cedarwood, and ylang-ylang.

Always check for contraindications, as some oils aren't suitable for use during pregnancy, for example.

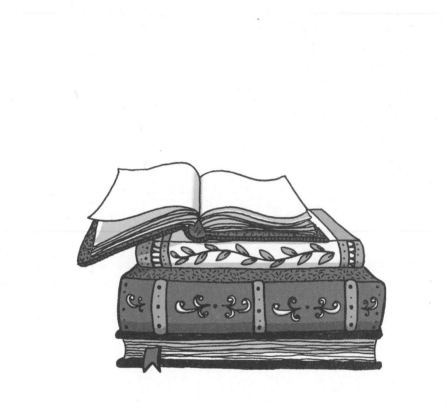

Conclusion

So there you have it!

Two hundred and twenty-two wide-ranging tips and tricks that I hope you've found interesting, enlightening, and most of all useful in helping you to enjoy better, more restful—and yes, blissful—sleep. I trust, too, that the book has made you realize that sleep is not the enemy, and that if you give it a fair and fighting chance by trying some of the calming strategies, wind-down tricks, and life tweaks that fill these pages, it can, and will, prevail over wakefulness.

Lastly, I hope that having all this information at your fingertips will make you feel more in control and convince you that—like everyone, everywhere—you have the power within you to sleep well and change your life for the better.

Thank you for reading my book, and I wish you peaceful sleep—tonight and every night.

Acknowledgments

Thank you to Alistair, for supporting me—and always believing in me; to my boys Steffan and Lucas and my family for encouraging me in this endeavor; and to my friends for cheering me on and confirming my belief that there's a need for as much easily accessible help as possible when it comes to getting a good night's sleep.

Thanks to my agent, Jennifer Christie, from Graham Maw Christie for her much-appreciated enthusiasm, humor, expert insight, and hard work (see you on the tennis court some time!); to Anna Steadman for commissioning the book and being a pleasure to work with; and to Jillian Young, Jillian Stewart, the rights team, and everyone else at Piatkus and Little, Brown, for their positivity and for championing the book. Thank you to everyone at The Experiment for the North American edition. Thank you, too, to Dr. Sarah Brewer and Lisa Artis for their kind words, and to Ruth Craddock for her charming illustrations.

References

Foreword

1. Christer Hublin et al., "Sleep and Mortality: A Population-Based 22-Year Follow-up Study," *Sleep* 30, no. 10 (2007): 1245–53, ncbi.nlm.nih.gov/pubmed/17969458.

Chapter 1: Before-Bed Wind-Down Tips

1. Amit Green et al., "Evening Light Exposure to Computer Screens Disrupts Human Sleep, Biological Rhythms, and Attention Abilities," *Chronobiology International*, 34, no. 7 (2017), 855–65, doi.org/10.1080/07420528.2017.1324878.

2. Heather Cleland Woods and Holly Scott, "#Sleepyteens: Social Media Use in Adolescence Is Associated with Poor Sleep Quality, Anxiety, Depression and Low Self-Esteem," *Journal of Adolescence* 51 (August 2016): 41–49, doi.org/10.1016/j.adolescence.2016.05.008; Nikos Xanidis and Catherine M. Brignell, "The Association between the Use of Social Network Sites, Sleep Quality and Cognitive

Function during the Day," *Computers in Human Behavior*, 55, part A (2016): 121–6, doi.org/10.1016/j.chb.2015.09.004.

3. See rsph.org.uk/uploads/assets/uploaded/ d125b27c-0b62-41c5-a2c0155a8887cd01.pdf.

4. Laurence Bayer et al., "Rocking Synchronizes Brain Waves during a Short Nap," *Current Biology* 21, no. 12 (2011): R461–R462, doi.org/ 10.1016/j.cub.2011.05.012.

5. J. A. Horne and B. S. Shackell, "Slow-Wave Sleep Elevations after Body Heating: Proximity to Sleep and Effects of Aspirin," *Sleep* 10, no. 4 (1987): 383–92.

6. Adam W. Hanley et al., "Washing Dishes to Wash the Dishes: Brief Instruction in an Informal Mindfulness Practice," *Mindfulness* 6, no. 5: 1095, dx.doi.org/10.1007/s12671-014-0360-9.

7. Emre Selcuk et al., "Perceived Partner Responsiveness Predicts Better Sleep Quality through Lower Anxiety," *Social Psychological and Personality Science* 8, no. 1 (2016): 83–92.

8. David Lewis, Galaxy Stress Research, Mindlab International, Sussex University, UK, 2009.

9. Anna Ejindu, "The Effects of Foot and Facial Massage on Sleep Induction, Blood Pressure, Pulse and Respiratory Rate: Crossover Pilot Study," *Complementary Therapies in Clinical Practice* 13, no. 4 (2007), 266–75, doi.org/10.1016/j.ctcp.2007.03.008.

10. Winai Sayorwan et al., "The Effects of Lavender Oil Inhalation on Emotional States, Autonomic Nervous System, and Brain Electrical Activity," *Journal of the Medical Association of Thailand* 95 (2012): 598–606.

11. George T. Lewith, Anthony Dean Godfrey, and Philip Prescott, "A Single-Blinded, Randomized Pilot Study Evaluating the Aroma of *Lavandula augustifolia* as a Treatment for Mild Insomnia," *Journal of Alternative and Complementary Medicine* 11, no. 4 (2005): 631–37.

12. I. M. McIntyre et al., "Human Melatonin Suppression by Light Is Intensity Dependent," *Journal of Pineal Research* 6, no. 2 (1989): 149–56, doi.org/10.1111/j.1600-079x.1989.tb00412.x.

13. Liese Exelmans and Jan Van den Bulck, "Binge Viewing, Sleep, and the Role of Pre-Sleep Arousal," *Journal of Clinical Sleep Medicine* 13, no. 8 (2017): 1001–8.

14. Elke Vlemincx, Ilse Van Diest, and Omer Van den Bergh, "A Sigh of Relief or a Sigh to Relieve: The Psychological and Physiological Relief Effect of Deep Breaths," *Physiology & Behavior* 165 (October 2016): 127–35, doi.org/10.1016/j.physbeh.2016.07.004.

15. László Harmat, Johanna Takács, and Róbert Bódizs, "Music Improves Sleep Quality in Students," *Journal of Advanced Nursing* 62, no. 3 (2008): 327–35, doi.org/10.1111/j.1365-2648.2008.04602.x.

16. Emma Barratt and Nick Davis, "Autonomous Sensory Meridian Response (ASMR): A Flow-Like Mental State," *PeerJ* 3, no. 2 (2015): e851, doi.org/10.7717/peerj.851.

17. Giulia Lara Poerio et al., "More Than a Feeling: Autonomous Sensory Meridian Response (ASMR) Is Characterized by Reliable Changes in Affect and Physiology," *PLoS ONE* 13, no. 6 (2018): e0196645, doi.org/10.1371/journal.pone.0196645.

18. Emi Morita et al., "A Before and After Comparison of the Effects of Forest Walking on the Sleep of a Community-Based Sample of People with Sleep Complaints," *Biopsychosocial Medicine* 5 (2011): e13, dx.doi.org/10.1186%2F1751-0759-5-13.

19. Michael K. Scullin et. al, "The Effects of Bedtime Writing on Difficulty Falling Asleep: A Polysomnographic Study Comparing To-Do Lists and Completed Activity Lists," *Journal of Experimental Psychology: General* 147, no. 1 (2018): 139–46, dx.doi.org/10.1037/xge0000374.

20. Mohsen Adib-Hajbaghery and Seyedeh Nesa Mousavi, "The Effects of Chamomile Extract on Sleep Quality among Elderly People: A Clinical Trial," *Complementary Therapies in Medicine*, 35 (2017): 109–14, doi.org/10.1016/j.ctim.2017.09.010.

21. Shao-Min Chang and Chung-Hey Chen, "Effects of an Intervention with Drinking Chamomile Tea on Sleep Quality and Depression in Sleep Disturbed Postnatal Women: A Randomized Controlled Trial," *Journal of Advanced Nursing* 72, no. 2 (2016), 306–15, doi.org/ 10.1111/jan.12836.

22. Michihito Igaki et al., "Effects of Bedtime Periocular and Posterior Cervical Cutaneous Warming on Sleep Status in Adult Male Subjects: A Preliminary Study," *Sleep and Biological Rhythms* 16, no. 1 (2018), 77–84, doi.org/10.1007/s41105-017-0129-3.

23. Bayer, "Rocking," R461–R462.

24. Ravindra Pattanashetty et al., "Practitioners of Vipassana Meditation Exhibit Enhanced Slow-Wave Sleep and REM Sleep States across Different Age Groups," *Sleep and Biological Rhythms* 8, no. 1 (2010): 34–41, doi.org/10.1111/j.1479-8425.2009.00416.x.

25. Britta K. Hölzel et al., "Mindfulness Practice Leads to Increases in Regional Brain Gray Matter Density," *Psychiatry Research* 191, no. 1 (2011): 36–43, doi.org/10.1016/j.pscychresns.2010.08.006.

26. G. A. Tooley et al., "Acute Increases in Night-Time Plasma Melatonin Levels Following a Period of Meditation," *Biological Psychology* 53, no. 1 (2000): 69–78, doi.org/10.1016/ s0301-0511(00)00035-1.

27. Rita W. Law, "An Analogue Study of Loving-Kindness Meditation as a Buffer against Social Stress," PhD diss., University of Arizona, 2011, repository.arizona.edu/handle/10150/145398.

28. Juan M. Manzaneque et al., "Serum Cytokines, Mood and Sleep after a Qigong Program: Is Qigong an Effective Psychobiological Tool?" *Journal of Health Psychology* 14, no. 1 (2009): 60–67, doi.org/10.1177/1359105308097946.

29. Shelley S. Tworoger et al., "Effects of a Yearlong Moderate-Intensity Exercise and a Stretching Intervention on Sleep Quality in Postmenopausal Women," *Sleep* 26, no. 7 (November 2003): 830–36.

30. Joannes Hallegraeff et al., "Stretching before Sleep Reduces the Frequency and Severity of Nocturnal Leg Cramps in Older Adults: A Randomised Trial," *Journal of Physiotherapy* 58, no. 1 (2012): 17–22; Mansooreh Aliasgharpour et al., "The Effect of Stretching Exercises on Severity of Restless Legs Syndrome in Patients on Hemodialysis," *Asian Journal of Sports Medicine* 7, no. 2 (2016): e31001.

31. Jyoti Arora, "Immediate Benefits of Om Chanting on Blood Pressure and Pulse Rate in Uncomplicated Moderate Hypertensive Subjects," *National Journal of Physiology, Pharmacy and Pharmacology* 8, no. 8 (2018): 1162–65, dx.doi.org/10.5455/njppp.2018.8.0413425042018.

32. Bangalore G Kalyani et al., "Neurohemodynamic Correlates of 'OM' Chanting: A Pilot Functional Magnetic Resonance Imaging Study," *International Journal of Yoga* 4, no. 1 (2011): 3–6.

Chapter 2: Mind Tricks

1. Alex M. Wood et al., "Gratitude Influences Sleep through the Mechanism of Pre-Sleep Cognitions," *Journal of Psychosomatic Research* 66, no. 1 (2009): 43–48, doi.org/10.1016/j.jpsychores.2008.09.002; Nancy Digdon and Amy Koble, "Effects of Constructive Worry, Imagery Distraction, and Gratitude Interventions on Sleep Quality: A Pilot Trial," *Applied Psychology: Health and Well-Being* 3, no. 2 (2011): 193–206, doi.org/10.1111/j.1758-0854.2011.01049.x.

2. Alexander James Kirkham, Julian Michael Breeze, and Paloma Marí-Beffa, "The Impact of Verbal Instructions on Goal-Directed Behavior," *Acta Psychologica* 139, no. 1 (2012): 212–19, doi.org/10.1016/j.actpsy.2011.09.016.

3. Allison G. Harvey, "The Attempted Suppression of Presleep Cognitive Activity in Insomnia," *Cognitive Therapy and Research* 27 (2003): 593–602, doi.org/10.1023/A:1026322310019.

4. Niall M. Broomfield and Colin A. Espie, "Initial Insomnia and Paradoxical Intention: An Experimental Investigation of Putative Mechanisms Using Subjective and Actigraphic Measurement of Sleep," *Behavioural and Cognitive Psychotherapy* 31, no. 3 (2003): 313–24, doi.org/10.1017/S1352465803003060.

5. Allison G. Harvey and Suzanna Payne (2002), "The Management of Unwanted Pre-Sleep Thoughts in Insomnia: Distraction with Imagery versus General Distraction," *Behaviour Research and Therapy* 40, no. 3 (2002): 267–77, doi.org/10.1016/s0005-7967(01)00012-2.

6. J. Nelson and Allison G. Harvey, "Pre-Sleep Imagery under the Microscope: A Comparison of Patients with Insomnia and Good Sleepers," *Behaviour Research and Therapy*, 41, no. 3 (2003): 273–84, doi.org/10.1016/S0005-7967(02)00010-4.

7. Stephen N. Haynes, Augustus Adams, and Michael Franzen, "The Effects of Pre-Sleep Stress on Sleep-Onset Insomnia," *Journal of Abnormal Psychology* 90, no. 6 (1981): 601–6, psycnet.apa.org/doi/10.1037/0021-843X.90.6.601.

8. H. Lai and M. Good, "Music Improves Sleep Quality in Older Adults," *Journal of Advanced Nursing* 49 (2005): 234–44, doi.org/10.1111/j.1365-2648.2004.03281.x.

9. Aviva Berkovich-Ohana et al., "Repetitive Speech Elicits Widespread Deactivation in the Human Cortex: The 'Mantra' Effect?" *Brain and Behavior* 5, no. 7 (2015): e00346, dx.doi.org/10.1002%2Fbrb3.346.

10. Matthew D. Lieberman et al., "Putting Feelings into Words," *Psychological Science* 18, no. 5 (2007): 421–28, doi.org/ 10.1111/j.1467- 9280.2007.01916.x.

11. Katharina Kircanski, Matthew D. Lieberman, and Michelle G. Craske, "Feelings into Words: Contributions of Language to Exposure Therapy," *Psychological Science* 23, no. 10 (2012): 1086–91, doi.org/10.1177/0956797612443830.

12. Jung Hwan Lee, Sun Yong Chung, and Jong Woo Kim, "A Comparison of Emotional Freedom Techniques, Insomnia (EFT- I) and Sleep Hygiene Education (SHE) for Insomnia in a Geriatric Population: A Randomized Controlled Trial," *Energy Psychology Journal* 7, no. 1 (2015): 22–29.

13. Jason C. Ong et al., "A Randomized Controlled Trial of Mindfulness Meditation for Chronic Insomnia," *Sleep* 37, no. 9 (2014): 1553–63, doi.org/10.5665/sleep.4010.

14. Cassandra D. Gould van Praag et al., "Mind-Wandering and Alterations to Default-Mode Network Connectivity when Listening to Naturalistic versus Artificial Sounds," *Scientific Reports* 7 (2017): 45273, doi.org/10.1038/srep45273.

15. American Academy of Sleep Medicine, "Cooling the Brain during Sleep May Be a Natural and Effective Treatment for Insomnia," *ScienceDaily*, June 13, 2011, sciencedaily.com/ releases/2011/06/110613093502.htm.

16. Kelly Glazer Baron et al., "Orthosomnia: Are Some Patients Taking the Quantified Self Too Far?" *Journal of Clinical Sleep Medicine* 13, no. 2 (2017): 351–54.

17. Kenneth L. Lichstein, "Insomnia Identity," *Behaviour Research and Therapy* 97 (2017): 230–41.

18. Nicole K. Y. Tang and Allison G. Harvey, "Correcting Distorted Perception of Sleep in Insomnia: A Novel Behavioural Experiment?" *Behaviour Research and Therapy* 42, no. 1 (2004): 27–39.

19. Gail Elliott Patricolo et al., "Beneficial Effects of Guided Imagery or Clinical Massage on the Status of Patients in a Progressive Care Unit," *Critical Care Nursing* 37, no. 1 (2017): 62–65, doi.org/10.4037/ccn2017282.

20. Melissa J. Ree et al., "Attempts to Control Unwanted Thoughts in the Night: Development of the Thought Control Questionnaire Insomnia Revised (TCQI-R)," *Behaviour Research and Therapy* 43, no. 8 (2005): 985–98, doi.org/10.1016/j.brat.2004.07.003; Les A. Gellis and Aesoon Park, "Nighttime Thought Control Strategies and Insomnia Severity," *Cognitive Therapy and Research* 37, no. 2 (2013): 383–89.

21. Jason S. Moser et al., "Third-Person Self-Talk Facilitates Emotion Regulation without Engaging Cognitive Control: Converging Evidence from ERP and fMRI," *Scientific Reports* 7 (2017): 4519, doi.org/10.1038/s41598-017-04047-3.

22. Maren Jasmin Cordi, Angelika A. Schlarb, and Björn Rasch, "Deepening Sleep by Hypnotic Suggestion," *Sleep* 37, no. 6 (2014): 1143–52, doi.org/10.5665/sleep.3778.

Chapter 3: Bedroom Tricks

1. B. H. Jacobson, A. Boolani, and D. B. Smith, "Changes in Back Pain, Sleep Quality, and Perceived Stress after Introduction of New Bedding Systems," *Journal of Chiropractic Medicine* 8, no. 1 (2009): 1–8, doi.org/10.1016/j.jcm.2008.09.002.

2. Mi Yang Jeon et al., "Improving the Quality of Sleep with an Optimal Pillow: A Randomized, Comparative Study," *Tohoku Journal of Experimental Medicine* 233, no. 3 (2014): 183–88, doi.org/10.1620/tjem.233.183.

3. Salma I. Patel et al., "The Effect of Dogs on Human Sleep in the Home Sleep Environment," *Mayo Clinic Proceedings* 92, no. 9 (2017): 1368–72.

4. National Sleep Foundation, "Bedroom Poll: Study of Findings," November 1, 2010, sleepfoundation.org/sites/default/files/ inline-files/NSF_Bedroom_Poll_Report.pdf.

5. Nelly A. Papalambros et al., "Acoustic Enhancement of Sleep Slow Oscillations and Concomitant Memory Improvement in Older Adults," *Frontiers in Human Neuroscience* 11 (2017): 109, doi.org/ 10.3389/fnhum.2017.00109.

6. Luigi Taranto Montemurro et al., "Effect of Background Noise on Sleep Quality," *Sleep* 40, suppl. 1 (2017): A146–A147, doi.org/ 10.1093/sleepj/zsx050.393.

7. Rochelle Ackerley, Gaby Badre, and Håkan Olausson, "Positive Effects of a Weighted Blanket on Insomnia," *Journal of Sleep Medicine and Disorders* 2, no. 3 (2015): 1022.

8. Kingston University London, "Messy Bedroom Could Spell End for Creepy Crawlies," January 17, 2005, kingston.ac.uk/news/ archive/2005/january/ 17-messy-bedroom-could-spell-end-for-creepy-crawlies.

9. Harumi Ikei, Chorong Song, and Yoshifumi Miyazaki, "Physiological Effects of Touching Wood," *International Journal of Environmental Research and Public Health* 14, no. 7 (2017): 801, doi.org/10.3390/ijerph14070801.

10. Magdalena Van den Berg et al., "Autonomic Nervous System Responses to Viewing Green and Built Settings: Differentiating between Sympathetic and Parasympathetic Activity," *International Journal of Environmental Research and Public Health* 12, no. 12 (2015): 15860–74.

11. B. C. Wolverton et al., "A Study of Interior Landscape Plants for Indoor Air Pollution Abatement," NASA, July 1989, archive.org/details/nasa_techdoc_19930072988.

12. St. Lawrence University, "Student-Faculty Sleep Research Published, Presented," June 10, 2015, stlawu.edu/news/student-faculty-sleep-research-published-presented.

Chapter 4: Food and Drink Tips

1. Stephen J. Edwards et al., "Spicy Meal Disturbs Sleep: An Effect of Thermoregulation?" *International Journal of Psychophysiology* 13, no. 2 (1992): 97–100, doi.org/10.1016/0167-8760(92)90048-G.

2. Marie-Pierre St-Onge et al., "Fiber and Saturated Fat Are Associated with Sleep Arousals and Slow Wave Sleep," *Journal of Clinical Sleep Medicine* 12, no. 1 (2016): 19–24, doi.org/10.5664/jcsm.5384.

3. Ibid.

4. Aric A. Prather et al., "Short and Sweet: Associations between Self- Reported Sleep Duration and Sugar-Sweetened Beverage Consumption among Adults in the United States," *Sleep Health* 2, no. 4 (2016): 272–76, doi.org/10.1016/j.sleh.2016.09.007.

5. Shubhroz Gill and Satchidananda Panda, "A Smartphone App Reveals Erratic Diurnal Eating Patterns in Humans That Can Be Modulated for Health Benefits," *Cell Metabolism* 22, no. 5 (2015): 789–98, doi.org/10.1016/j.cmet.2015.09.005.

6. Andreas Nievergelt et al., "Identification of Serotonin 5-HT1A Receptor Partial Agonists in Ginger," *Bioorganic and Medicinal Chemistry* 18, no. 9 (2010): 3345–51, doi.org/10.1016/j.bmc.2010.02.062; K. Chandrasekhar, Jyoti Kapoor, and Sridhar Anishetty," A Prospective, Randomized Double-Blind, Placebo-Controlled Study of Safety and Efficacy of a High-Concentration Full-Spectrum Extract of Ashwagandha Root

in Reducing Stress and Anxiety in Adults," *Indian Journal of Psychological Medicine* 34, no. 3 (2012): 255–62.

7. Essra Noorwali et al., "The Relationship between Sleep Duration and Fruit/Vegetable Intakes in UK Adults: A Cross-Sectional Study from the National Diet and Nutrition Survey," *BMJ Open* 8, no. 4 (2018): e020810, dx.doi.org/10.1136/bmjopen-2017-020810.

8. Robert S. Thompson et al., "Dietary Prebiotics and Bioactive Milk Fractions Improve NREM Sleep, Enhance REM Sleep Rebound and Attenuate the Stress-Induced Decrease in Diurnal Temperature and Gut Microbial Alpha Diversity," *Frontiers in Behavioral Neuroscience* 10, (2016): 240, doi.org/10.3389/fnbeh.2016.00240.

9. St-Onge, "Fiber and Saturated Fat."

10. Irshaad O. Ebrahim et al., "Alcohol and Sleep I: Effects on Normal Sleep," *Alcoholism: Clinical and Experimental Research* 37, no. 4 (2013): 539–49, doi.org/10.1111/acer.12006.

11. Russel J. Reiter et al., , "Melatonin in Walnuts: Influence on Levels of Melatonin and Total Antioxidant Capacity of Blood," *Nutrition* 21, no. 9 (2005): 920–24.

12. Michael D. Drennan et al., "Potassium Affects Actigraph-Identified Sleep," *Sleep* 14, no. 4 (1991): 357–60.

13. Stephen Bent et al., "Valerian for Sleep: A Systematic Review and Meta-Analysis," *American Journal of Medicine* 119, no. 12 (2006): 1005–12.

14. Katri Peuhkuri, Nora Jaatinen, and Riitta Korpela, "Diet Promotes Sleep Duration and Quality," *Nutrition Research* 32, no. 5 (2012): 309–19; C. Markus, L. Jonkman, J. Lammers, N. Deutz, M. Messer, N. Rigtering (2005), C. Rob Markus et al., "Evening Intake of Alpha-Lactalbumin Increases Plasma Tryptophan Availability and Improves Morning Alertness and Brain Measures of Attention," *American Journal of Clinical Nutrition* 81, no. 5: 1026–33.

15. B. Spring, "Recent Research on the Behavioral Effects of Tryptophan and Carbohydrate," *Nutrition and Health* 3, nos. 1–2 (1984): 55–67.

16. Jack N. Losso et al., "Pilot Study of the Tart Cherry Juice for the Treatment of Insomnia and Investigation of Mechanisms," *American Journal of Therapeutics* 25, no. 2 (2018): e194–e201, doi.org/10.1097/MJT.0000000000000584.

17. Hsiao-Han Lin et al., "Effect of Kiwifruit Consumption on Sleep Quality in Adults with Sleep Problems," *Asia Pacific Journal of Clinical Nutrition* 20, no. 2 (2011): 169–74.

18. Keiko Unno et al., "Reduced Stress and Improved Sleep Quality Caused by Green Tea Are Associated with a Reduced Caffeine Content," *Nutrients* 9, no. 7 (2017): 777, doi.org/10.3390/nu9070777; Keiko Unno et al., "Ingestion of Green Tea with Lowered Caffeine Improves Sleep Quality of the Elderly via Suppression of Stress," *Journal of Clinical Biochemistry and Nutrition* 61, no. 3 (2017): 210–16, doi.org/10.3164/jcbn.17-6.

19. Behnood Abbasi et al., "The Effect of Magnesium Supplementation on Primary Insomnia in the Elderly: A Double-Blind Placebo-Controlled Clinical Trial," *Journal of Research in Medical Sciences* 17, no. 12 (2012): 1161–69.

20. A. Ngan and Russell Conduit, "A Double-Blind, Placebo-Controlled Investigation of the Effects of *Passiflora incarnata* (Passionflower) Herbal Tea on Subjective Sleep Quality," *Phytotherapy Research* 25, no. 8 (2011): 1153–59, doi.org/10.1002/ptr.3400.

21. Anita Lill Hansen et al., "Fish Consumption, Sleep, Daily Functioning, and Heart Rate Variability," *Journal of Clinical Sleep Medicine* 10, no. 5 (2014): 567–75, doi.org/10.5664/jcsm.3714.

Chapter 5: Body Tricks

1. Stephen R. Arnott, Anthony Singhal, and Melvyn A. Goodale, "An Investigation of Auditory Contagious Yawning," *Cognitive, Affective, and Behavioral Neuroscience* 9, no. 3 (2009): 335–42; Robert R. Provine, "Yawning as a Stereotyped Action Pattern and Releasing Stimulus," *Ethology* 72, no. 2 (1986): 109–22.

2. Nahid Golmakani et al., "Comparing the Effects of Progressive Muscle Relaxation and Guided Imagery on Sleep Quality in Primigravida Women Referring to Mashhad Health Care Centers—1393," *Journal of Midwifery and Reproductive Health* 3, no. 2 (2015): 335–42; Nuray Dayapoğlu and Mehtap Tan, "Evaluation of the Effect of Progressive Relaxation Exercises on Fatigue and Sleep Quality in Patients with Multiple Sclerosis," *Journal of Alternative and Complementary Medicine* 18, no. 10 (2012): 983–87, doi.org/10.1089/acm.2011.0390; Zümrüt Akgün Sahin and Nuray Dayapoğlu, "Effect of Progressive Relaxation Exercises on Fatigue and Sleep Quality in Patients with Chronic Obstructive Lung Disease (COPD)," *Complementary Therapies in Clinical Practice* 21, no. 4 (2015): 277–81, doi.org/10.1016/j.ctcp.2015.10.002.

3. Kathleen C. Light, Karen M. Grewen, and Janet A. Amico, "More Frequent Partner Hugs and Higher Oxytocin Levels Are Linked to Lower Blood Pressure and Heart Rate in Premenopausal Women," *Biological Psychology* 69, no. 1 (2005): 5–21, doi.org/10.1016/j.biopsycho.2004.11.002.

4. Kurt Kräuchi et al., "Physiology: Warm Feet Promote the Rapid Onset of Sleep," *Nature* 401, no. 6748 (1999): 36–37.

5. Yelin Ko and Joo-Young Lee, "Effects of Feet Warming Using Bed Socks on Sleep Quality and Thermoregulatory Responses in a Cool Environment," *Journal of Physiological Anthropology* 37, no. 13 (2018), doi.org/10.1186/s40101-018-0172-z.

6. Melodee Harris, Kathy Culpepper Richards, and Victoria T. Grando, "The Effects of Slow- Stroke Back Massage on Minutes of Nighttime Sleep in Persons with Dementia and Sleep Disturbances in the Nursing Home: A Pilot Study," *Journal of Holistic Nursing* 30, no. 4 (2012): 255–63, doi.org/10.1177%2F0898010112455948.

7. Tara L. Kraft and Sarah D. Pressman, "Grin and Bear It: The Influence of Manipulated Facial Expression on the Stress Response," *Psychological Science* 23, no. 11 (2012): 1372–78, doi.org/10.1177/0956797612445312.

8. Vanessa Ieto et al., "Effects of Oropharyngeal Exercises on Snoring," *CHEST* 148, no. 3 (2015): 683–91.

9. Rong fang Hu et al., "Effects of Earplugs and Eye Masks on Nocturnal Sleep, Melatonin and Cortisol in a Simulated Intensive Care Unit Environment," *Critical Care* 14, no. 2 (2010): R66, doi.org/10.1186/cc8965; Fatemeh Mashayekhi et al., "The Effect of Eye Mask on Sleep Quality in Patients of Coronary Care Unit," *Sleep Science* 6, no. 3 (2013): 108–11.

10. Victoria Bion et al., "Reducing Sound and Light Exposure to Improve Sleep on the Adult Intensive Care Unit: An Inclusive Narrative Review," *Journal of the Intensive Care Society* 19, no. 2 (2017): 138–46, doi.org/10.1177/1751143717740803.

11. Joseph de Koninck, Pierre Gagnon, and Serge Lallier, "Sleep Positions in the Young Adult and Their Relationship with the Subjective Quality of Sleep," *Sleep* 6, no. 1 (1983): 52–59, doi.org/10.1093/sleep/6.1.52.

12. Vera Abeln et al., "Brainwave Entrainment for Better Sleep and Post-Sleep State of Young Elite Soccer Players: A Pilot Study," *European Journal of Sport Science* 14, no. 5 (2014): 393–402, doi.org/10.1080/17461391.2013.819384; Rene Pierre Le Scouarnec et al., "Use of Binaural Beat Tapes for Treatment of Anxiety: A Pilot Study

of Tape Preference and Outcomes," *Alternative Therapies in Health and Medicine* 7, no. 1 (January 2001): 58–63; R. Padmanabhan, A. J. Hildreth, and D. Laws, "A Prospective, Randomized, Controlled Study Examining Binaural Beat Audio and Pre-Operative Anxiety in Patients Undergoing General Anaesthesia for Day-Case Surgery," *Anaesthesia* 60, no. 9 (2005): 874–77, doi.org/10.1111/j.1365-2044.2005.04287.x.

13. Roy J. E. M. Raymann, Dick F. Swaab, and Eus J. W. Van Someren, "Cutaneous Warming Promotes Sleep Onset," *American Journal of Physiology, Regulatory, Integrative and Comparative Physiology* 288, no. 6 (2005): R1589–R1597.

14. Rick Hanson, "Relaxed and Contented: Activating the Parasympathetic Wing of Your Nervous System," WiseBrain.org, 2007, wisebrain.org/ParasympatheticNS.pdf.

15. Yuchi Wu et al., "Auricular Acupressure Helps Improve Sleep Quality for Severe Insomnia in Maintenance Hemodialysis Patients: A Pilot Study," *Journal of Alternative and Complementary Medicine* 20, no 5 (2014): 356–63; Yi-Li Ko, Shih-Chi Lin, and Pi-Chu Lin, "Effect of Auricular Acupressure for Postpartum Insomnia: An Uncontrolled Clinical Trial," *Journal of Clinical Nursing* 25, no. 3 (2016), 332–39, doi.org/10.1111/jocn.13053; Nam Hyun Cha, Yi Kyun Park, and Sohyune R. Sok, "Effects of Auricular Acupressure Therapy on Stress and Sleep Disturbance of Middle-Aged Women in South Korea," *Holistic Nursing Practice* 31, no. 2 (2017): 102–9, dx.doi.org/10.1097/HNP.0000000000000372.

16. Donna Lamke, Anita Catlin, and Michelle Mason-Chadd, "'Not Just a Theory': The Relationship between Jin Shin Jyutsu® Self-Care Training for Nurses and Stress, Physical Health, Emotional Health, and Caring Efficacy," *Journal of Holistic Nursing* 32, no. 44 (2014): 278–89, dx.doi.org/10.1177/0898010114531906.

17. L. C. Katz, R. Just, and D.O. Castell, "Body Position Affects Recumbent Postprandial Reflux," *Journal of Clinical*

Gastroenterology 18, no. 4 (1994): 280–83; M. A. Van Herwaarden et al., "Effect of Different Recumbent Positions on Postprandial Gastroesophageal Reflux in Normal Subjects," *American Journal of Gastroenterology* 95, no. 10 (2000): 2731–36; R. M. Khoury et al., "Influence of Spontaneous Sleep Positions on Nighttime Recumbent Reflux in Patients with Gastroesophageal Reflux Disease," *American Journal of Gastroenterology* 94, no. 8 (1999): 2069–73; L. C. Katz, R. Just, and D. O. Castell, "Body Position Affects Recumbent Postprandial Reflux," *Journal of Clinical Gastroenterology* 18, no. 4 (1994): 280–83; M. A. Van Herwaarden et al., "Effect of Different Recumbent Positions on Postprandial Gastroesophageal Reflux in Normal Subjects," *American Journal of Gastroenterology* 95, no. 10 (2000): 2731–36; R. M. Khoury et al., "Influence of Spontaneous Sleep Positions on Nighttime Recumbent Reflux in Patients with Gastroesophageal Reflux Disease," *American Journal of Gastroenterology* 94, no. 8 (1999): 2069–73.

Chapter 6: Breathing Tricks

1. Ananda Balayogi Bhavanani, Madanmohan, and Zeena Sanjay, "Immediate Effect of Chandra Nadi Pranayama (Left Unilateral Forced Nostril Breathing) on Cardiovascular Parameters in Hypertensive Patients," *International Journal of Yoga* 5, no. 2 (2012): 108–11, doi.org/10.4103/0973-6131.98221.

2. Sukhdev Singh, Vishaw Gaurav, and Ved Parkash, "Effects of a 6-Week Nadi-Shodhana Pranayama Training on Cardiopulmonary Parameters," *Journal of Physical Education and Sports Management* 2, no. 4 (2011): 44–47.

3. Wang Shu- Zhen et al., "Effect of Slow Abdominal Breathing Combined with Biofeedback on Blood Pressure and Heart Rate Variability in Prehypertension," *Journal of Alternative and Complementary Medicine* 16, no. 10 (2010): 1039–45, doi.org/10.1089/acm.2009.0577.

4. Chacko N. Joseph et al., "Slow Breathing Improves Arterial Baroreflex Sensitivity and Decreases Blood Pressure in Essential Hypertension," *Hypertension* 46 (2005): 714–18.

5. Keven Yackle et al., "Breathing Control Center Neurons That Promote Arousal in Mice," *Science* 355, no. 6332 (2017): 1411–15, doi.org/10.1126/science.aai7984.

Chapter 7: Daytime Tricks

1. Markus Jansson-Fröjmark, Marcus Lind, and Rikard Sunnhed, "Don't Worry, Be Constructive: A Randomized Controlled Feasibility Study Comparing Behaviour Therapy Singly and Combined with Constructive Worry for Insomnia," *British Journal of Clinical Psychology* 51, no. 2 (2012): 142–57, doi.org/10.1111/j.2044- 8260.2011.02018.x; Nancy Digdon and Amy Koble, "Effects of Constructive Worry, Imagery Distraction, and Gratitude Interventions on Sleep Quality: A Pilot Trial," *Applied Psychology: Health and Well-Being* 3, no. 2 (2011): 193–206, doi.org/10.1111/j.1758- 0854.2011.01049.x.

2. Colleen E. Carney and William F. Waters, "Effects of a Structured Problem-Solving Procedure on Pre-Sleep Cognitive Arousal in College Students with Insomnia," *Behavioral Sleep Medicine* 4, no. 1 (2006): 13–28, doi.org/10.1207/s15402010bsm0401_2.

3. M. Boubekri et al., "Impact of Windows and Daylight Exposure on Overall Health and Sleep Quality of Office Workers: A Case-Control Pilot Study," *Journal of Clinical Sleep Medicine* 10, no. 6 (2014): 603–11, doi.org/10.5664/jcsm.3780.

4. Chih-Hsiang Yang and David E. Conroy, "Momentary Negative Affect Is Lower during Mindful Movement Than while Sitting: An Experience-Sampling Study," *Psychology of Sport and Exercise* 37 (2018): 109–16, doi.org/10.1016/j.psychsport.2018.05.003.

5. David S. Black et al., "Mindfulness Meditation and Improvement in Sleep Quality and Daytime Impairment among Older Adults with Sleep Disturbances: A Randomized Clinical Trial," *JAMA Internal Medicine* 175, no. 4 (2015): 494–501, doi.org/10.1001/jamainternmed.2014.8081.

6. Judy Pa et al., "Effect of Exercise and Cognitive Activity on Self-Reported Sleep Quality in Community-Dwelling Older Adults with Cognitive Complaints: A Randomized Controlled Trial," *Journal of the American Geriatrics Society* 62, no. 12 (2014): 2319–26, doi.org/10.1111/jgs.13158.

7. Daniel T. C. Cox et al., "Doses of Neighborhood Nature: The Benefits for Mental Health of Living with Nature," *BioScience* 67, no. 2 (2017): 147–55, doi.org/10.1093/biosci/biw173.

8. Anthony D. Ong et al., "Linking Stable and Dynamic Features of Positive Affect to Sleep," *Annals of Behavioral Medicine* 46, no. 1 (2013): 52, doi.org/10.1007/s12160-013-9484-8.

9. Kimberly Y. Z. Forrest and Wendy L. Stuhldreher, "Prevalence and Correlates of Vitamin D Deficiency in US adults," *Sleep* 31, no. 1 (2011): 48–54, doi.org/10.1016/j.nutres.2010.12.001.

10. Mohammad Shahi Majid et al., "The Effect of Vitamin D Supplement on the Score and Quality of Sleep in 20–50 Year-Old People with Sleep Disorders Compared with Control Group," *Nutritional Neuroscience* 21, no. 1 (2017): 511–519, doi.org/10.1080/1028415X.2017.1317395.

11. National Institutes of Health: Office of Dietary Supplements, "Vitamin D: Fact Sheet for Health Professionals," U.S. Department of Health and Human Services, August 7, 2019, ods.od.nih.gov/factsheets/VitaminD-HealthProfessional.

12. J. A. Horne and A. Minard, "Sleep and Sleepiness Following a Behaviourally 'Active' Day," *Ergonomics* 28, no. 3 (1985), 567–75, doi.org/10.1080/00140138508963171.

13. Sabine Sonnentag, "Psychological Detachment from Work during Leisure Time and the Benefits of Mentally Disengaging from Work," *Current Directions in Psychological Science*, 21, no. 2 (2012): 114–18, doi.org/10.1177/0963721411434979; Cathleen Clerkin, Marian Ruderman, and Elena Svetieva, "Tired at Work: A Roadblock to Effective Leadership," Center for Creative Leadership, 2017, ccl.org/wp-content/uploads/2017/11/Tired-at-Work-Roadblock-to-effective-leadership-white-paper.pdf.

14. Caitlin A. Demsky et al., "Workplace Incivility and Employee Sleep: The Role of Rumination and Recovery Experiences," *Journal of Occupational Health Psychology* 24, no. 2 (2018): 228–40, doi.org/0.1037/ocp0000116.

15. Sabine Sonnentag and Charlotte Fritz, "The Recovery Experience Questionnaire: Development and Validation of a Measure for Assessing Recuperation and Unwinding from Work," *Journal of Occupational Health Psychology* 12, no. 3 (2007): 204–21, doi.org/10.1037/1076-8998.12.3.204.

16. Julianne Holt-Lunstad, Timothy B. Smith, and J. Bradley Layton, "Social Relationships and Mortality Risk: A Meta-Analytic Review," *PLoS Medicine* 7, no. 7 (2010): e1000316, doi.org/10.1371/journal.pmed.1000316.

17. Royette Tavernier, "Adolescents' Technology and Face-to-Face Time Use Predict Objective Sleep Outcomes," *Sleep Health* 3, no. 4 (2017): 276–83, doi.org/10.1016/j.sleh.2017.04.005.

18. Lianne M. Kurina et al., "Loneliness Is Associated with Sleep Fragmentation in a Communal Society," *Sleep* 34, no. 11 (2011): 1519–26, doi.org/10.5665/sleep.1390; John T. Cacioppo et al., "Loneliness and Health: Potential Mechanisms," *Psychosomatic Medicine* 64, no. 3 (2002): 407–17.

19. Jill Riley, Betsan Corkhill, and Clare Morris, "The Benefits of Knitting for Personal and Social Wellbeing in Adulthood: Findings from an International Survey," *British Journal of Occupational Therapy* 76, no. 2 (2013): 50–57.

20. Nancy A. Curry and Tim Kasser, "Can Coloring Mandalas Reduce Anxiety?" *Art Therapy* 22, no. 2 (2005), 81–85, doi.org/10.1080/07421656.2005.10129441; Jayde A. M. Flett et al., "Sharpen Your Pencils: Preliminary Evidence that Adult Coloring Reduces Depressive Symptoms and Anxiety," *Creativity Research Journal* 29, no. 4 (2017): 409–16, doi.org/10.1080/10400419.2017.1376505.

21. Ilana S. Hairston and Roni Shpitalni, "Procrastination Is Linked with Insomnia Symptoms: The Moderating Role of Morningness-Eveningness," *Personality and Individual Differences* 101 (2016): 50–56, doi.org/10.1016/j.paid.2016.05.031.

22. Hayan Lee, Sunho Kim, and Donghee Kim, "Effects of Exercise with or without Light Exposure on Sleep Quality and Hormone Responses," *Journal of Exercise Nutrition & Biochemistry* 18, no. 3 (2014): 293–99, doi.org/10.5717/jenb.2014.18.3.293.

23. Indrani Ganguly-Fitzgerald, Jeff Donlea, and Paul J. Shaw, "Waking Experience Affects Sleep Need in Drosophila," *Science* 313, no. 5794 (2006), 1775–81.

24. Kathryn J. Reid et al., "Aerobic Exercise Improves Self-Reported Sleep and Quality of Life in Older Adults with Insomnia," *Sleep Medicine* 11, no. 9 (2010): 934–40, doi.org/10.1016/j.sleep.2010.04.014.

Chapter 8: Tips for Taking the Stress out of Sleep

1. Hae-Jin Ko and Changho Youn, "Effects of Laughter Therapy on Depression, Cognition and Sleep among the Community-Dwelling Elderly," *Geriatrics & Gerontology International* 11, no. 3 (2011): 267–74, doi.org/10.1111/j.1447- 0594.2010.00680.x.

2. Hajime Kimata, "Laughter Elevates the Levels of Breast-Milk Melatonin," *Journal of Psychosomatic Research* 62, no. 6 (2007): 699–702.

3. Ellen R. Stothard et al., "Circadian Entrainment to the Natural Light-Dark Cycle across Seasons and the Weekend," *Current Biology* 27, no. 4 (2017): 508–13, doi.org/10.1016/j.cub.2016.12.041.

4. Arlener D. Turner, Christine E. Smith, and Jason C. Ong, "Is Purpose in Life Associated with Less Sleep Disturbance in Older Adults?" *Sleep Science and Practice* 1, no. 14 (2017), doi.org/10.1186/s41606-017-0015-6.

5. Arthur J. Spielman, Paul Saskin, and Michael J. Thorpy, "Treatment of Chronic Insomnia by Restriction of Time in Bed," *Sleep* 10, no. 1 (1987): 45–56.

6. Sat Bir Singh Khalsa, "Treatment of Chronic Insomnia with Yoga: A Preliminary Study with Sleep-Wake Diaries," *Applied Psychophysiology Biofeedback* 29, no. 4 (2004): 269–78, doi.org/10.1007/s10484-004-0387-0.

7. Paul D. Loprinzi and Bradley J. Cardinal, "Association between Objectively Measured Physical Activity and Sleep, NHANES 2005–2006," *Mental Health and Physical Activity* 4, no. 2 (2011): 65–69, doi.org/10.1016/j.mhpa.2011.08.001; Kathryn J. Reid et al., "Aerobic Exercise Improves Self-Reported Sleep and Quality of Life in Older Adults with Insomnia," *Sleep Medicine* 11, no. 9 (2010): 934–40, doi.org/10.1016/j.sleep.2010.04.014; José M. T. Bonardi et al., "Effect of Different Types of Exercise on Sleep Quality of Elderly Subjects," *Sleep Medicine* 25 (2016): 122–29, doi.org/10.1016/j.sleep.2016.06.025.

8. Helen Rockliff et al., "A Pilot Exploration of Heart Rate Variability and Salivary Cortisol Responses to Compassion-Focused Imagery," *Clinical Neuropsychiatry* 5, no. 3 (2008): 132–39.

9. Emi Morita et al., "A Before and After Comparison of the Effects of Forest Walking on the Sleep of a Community-Based Sample of People with Sleep Complaints," *Biopsychosocial Medicine* 5, no. 13 (2011), dx.doi.org/10.1186/1751-0759-5-13.

10. Sin-Ae Park et al., "Foliage Plants Cause Physiological and Psychological Relaxation as Evidenced by Measurements of Prefrontal Cortex Activity and Profile of Mood States," *HortScience* 51, no. 10 (2016): 1308–12; Chorong Song et al., "Physiological Effects of Viewing Fresh Red Roses," *Complementary Therapies in Medicine* 35 (2017): 78–84; Hiroko Ochiai et al., "Effects of Visual Stimulation with Bonsai Trees on Adult Male Patients with Spinal Cord Injury," *International Journal of Environmental Research and Public Health* 14, no. 9 (2017): 1017.

11. Ann Bowden, Ava Lorenc, and Nicola Robinson, "Autogenic Training as a Behavioural Approach to Insomnia: A Prospective Cohort Study," *Primary Health Care Research & Development* 13, no. 2 (2012): 175–85, doi.org/10.1017/S1463423611000181.

12. Tromholt Morten, "The Facebook Experiment: Quitting Facebook Leads to Higher Levels of Well-Being," *Cyberpsychology, Behavior, and Social Networking* 19, no. 11 (2016): 661–66.

13. Gloria Mark, Stephen Voida, and Armand Cardello, "'A Pace Not Dictated by Electrons': An Empirical Study of Work without Email," *Chi '12: Proceedings of the SIGCHI Conference on Human Factors in Computing Systems*, May 2012, pp. 555–64, doi.org/10.1145/2207676.2207754.

14. Martha E. Billings et al., "Relationship of Air Pollution to Sleep Disruption: The Multi-Ethnic Study of Atherosclerosis (MESA) Sleep and MESA-Air Studies," *American Journal of Respiratory and Critical Care Medicine* 195 (2017): A2930.

15. D. Warren Spence et al., "Acupuncture Increases Nocturnal Melatonin Secretion and Reduces Insomnia and Anxiety: A Preliminary Report," *Journal of Neuropsychiatry and Clinical Neurosciences* 16, no. 1 (2004): 19–28; Johannah L Shergis et al., "A Systematic Review of Acupuncture for Sleep Quality in People with Insomnia," *Complementary Therapies in Medicine* 26 (2016): 11–20.

16. David W. Wetter and Terry B. Young, "The Relation between Cigarette Smoking and Sleep Disturbance," *Preventive Medicine* 23, no. 3 (1994): 328–34.

17. Ravindra Kashyap, Lynette M. Hock, and Teri J. Bowman, "Higher Prevalence of Smoking in Patients Diagnosed as Having Obstructive Sleep Apnea," *Sleep and Breathing* 5, no. 4 (2001): 167–72, doi.org/10.1055/s-2001-18805.

18. Benedict W. Wheeler, Mathew White, Will Stahl-Timmins, Michael H. Depledge, "Does living by the coast improve health and wellbeing?" *Health & Place* 18, no. 5 (2012): 1198–1201, doi.org/10.1016/j.healthplace.2012.06.015.

19. Eleanor Ratcliffe, "Sleep, Mood, and Coastal Walking: Report Prepared for the National Trust," August 2015, nationaltrust.org.uk/ documents/sleep-mood-andcoastal-walking---a-report-by-eleanor-ratcliffe.pdf.

20. Ari Shechter et al., "Blocking Nocturnal Blue Light for Insomnia: A Randomized Controlled Trial," *Journal of Psychiatric Research* 96 (2018): 196–202.

21. Esther Yuet Ying Lau et al., "Sleep and Optimism: A Longitudinal Study of Bidirectional Causal Relationship and Its Mediating and Moderating Variables in a Chinese Student Sample," *Chronobiology International* 34, no. 3 (2017): 360–72, doi.org/10.1080/07420528.2016.1276071.

22. Julia K. Boehm and Laura D. Kubzansky, "The Heart's Content: The Association between Positive Psychological Well-Being and Cardiovascular Health," *Psychological Bulletin* 138, no. 4 (2012): 655–91.

23. James H. Fowler and Nicholas A. Christakis, "Dynamic Spread of Happiness in a Large Social Network: Longitudinal Analysis over 20 Years in the Framingham Heart Study," *BMJ* 337 (2008): a2338.

24. Eunhee Hwang and Sujin Shin, "The Effects of Aromatherapy on Sleep Improvement: A Systematic Literature Review and Meta-Analysis," *Journal of Alternative Complementary Medicine* 21, no. 2 (2015): 61–68; Ai Takeda, Emiko Watanuki, and Sachiyo Koyama, "Effects of Inhalation Aromatherapy on Symptoms of Sleep Disturbance in the Elderly with Dementia," *Evidence-Based Complementary and Alternative Medicine*, no. 4 (2017), doi.org/10.1155/2017/1902807; Suganya Panneerselvam, "Effectiveness of Aromatherapy in Insomnia," *International Journal of Innovative Pharmaceutical Sciences and Research* 5 (2017): 96–106, doi.org/10.21276/IJIPSR.2017.05.11.220; Ezgi Karadag et al., "Effects of Aromatherapy on Sleep Quality and Anxiety of Patients," *Nursing in Critical Care* 22, no. 2 (2017): 105–12, doi.org/10.1111/nicc.12198.

About the Author

KIM JONES is a freelance journalist specializing in health and well-being. She is a member of the Guild of Health Writers and writes for various national women's magazines and newspapers in the UK, including the *Daily Mirror*, the *Sunday Express Magazine*, *Woman's Weekly*, *Tesco Magazine*, and *Woman and Home*. Kim lives in Cardiff with her partner, their two sons, a cat, and cocker spaniel.